food intolerance
management plan

Dr Sue Shepherd, an Advanced Accredited Practising Dietitian and Accredited Nutritionist, specialises in the treatment of dietary intolerances. She has a Bachelor of Applied Science in Health Promotion, a Masters in Nutrition and Dietetics, and a PhD for her research into coeliac disease, the Low-FODMAP Diet, fructose malabsorption and irritable bowel syndrome. Sue, who has coeliac disease herself, lives and breathes gluten-free and low-FODMAP. For creating the Low-FODMAP Diet, a world-first scientifically proven diet for people with IBS, she was awarded the Dietitians Association of Australia's Annual Award for Achievement, and the Gastroenterological Society of Australia's Young Investigator Award. She is the author of five cookbooks for people with coeliac disease, fructose malabsorption and irritable bowel syndrome, and runs a private practice, Shepherd Works, where she treats people with these conditions. She is the consultant dietitian on medical national advisory committees for gastrointestinal conditions. She also works as a dietitian in Box Hill Hospital and in her own private practice called Shepherd Works, and as a senior lecturer and research scientist, working with Peter Gibson at Monash University's Eastern Health Clinical School. She is passionate about good nutrition and healthy bowels!

Dr Peter Gibson is Professor of Medicine at Monash University and Head of the Eastern Health Clinical School. He is the Executive Clinical Director of Specialty Medicine and Director of Gastroenterology and Hepatology for Eastern Health (which includes Box Hill Hospital). After completing his medical degree with first-class honours, he pursued training in gastroenterology at Melbourne's Alfred Hospital and the John Radcliffe Hospital in Oxford, UK. In 1985 he was awarded an MD for his work on immunology and the bowel. After three years as a Research Fellow at the Australian National University, he joined the Department of Medicine at the University of Melbourne and the Royal Melbourne Hospital, where he was later Deputy Director of Gastroenterology. In 2001, he moved to Box Hill Hospital. A past president of the Gastroenterological Society of Australia, Peter has a long-standing interest in the influence of diet on bowel health. He has an international reputation as both a physician and researcher for such conditions as inflammatory bowel disease, coeliac disease and irritable bowel syndrome. He was recently awarded the Distinguished Research Prize by the Gastroenterological Society of Australia. Peter now leads a Monash University research team of dietitians, scientists and clinicians who are continuing to refine and extend our knowledge of the Low-FODMAP Diet.

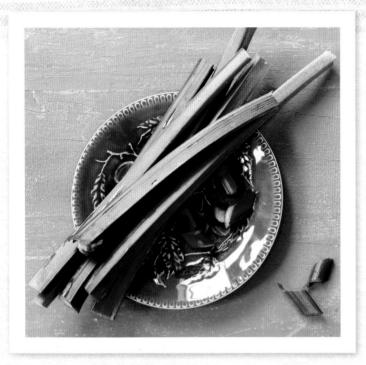
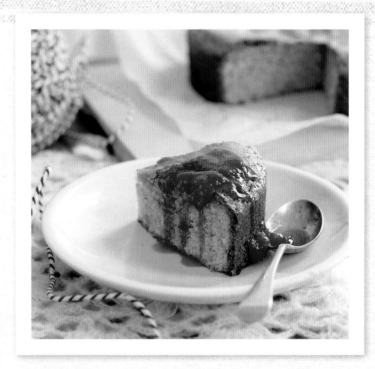
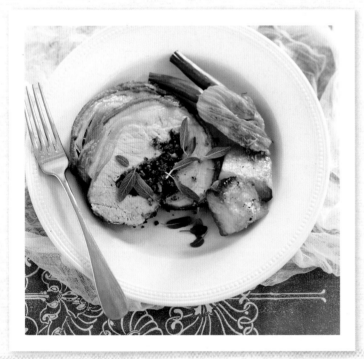
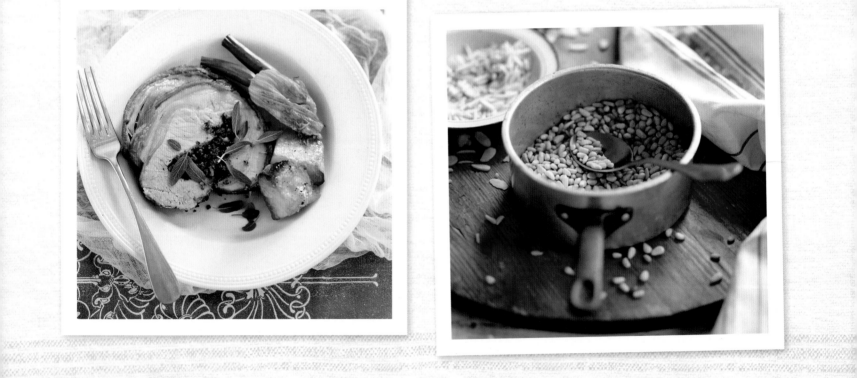

food intolerance
management plan

Dr Sue Shepherd & Dr Peter Gibson

Food photography by Mark O'Meara

VIKING
an imprint of
PENGUIN BOOKS

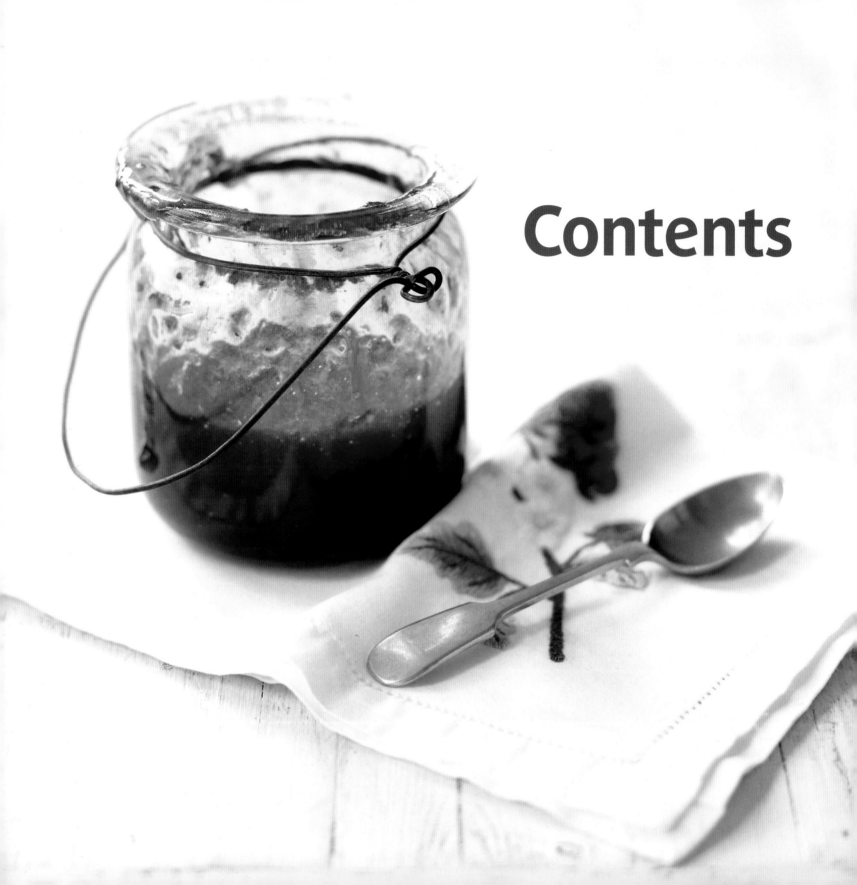

Contents

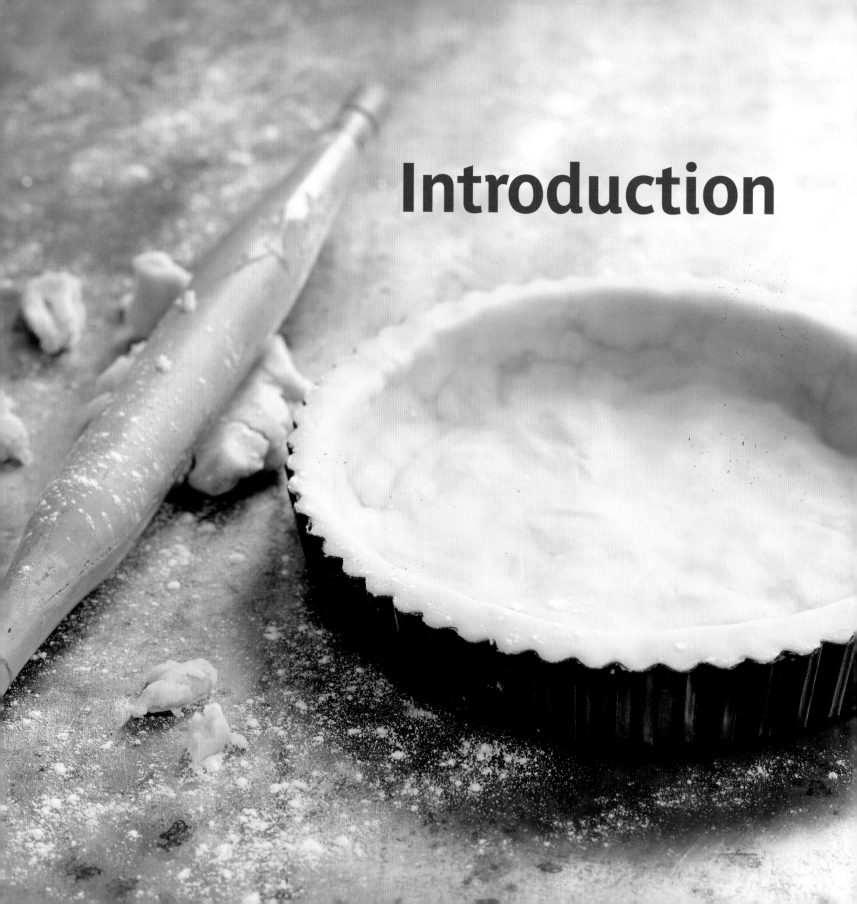

Introduction

IF YOU HAVE a food intolerance, suffer the symptoms of irritable bowel syndrome (IBS) – abdominal pain and bloating, excessive wind and diarrhoea or constipation or both – and are sick of feeling unwell, then this is the book for you. Our Low-FODMAP Diet for IBS sufferers has transformed the lives of lots of people and could work for you. We'll explain what low-FODMAP means (see page 23) and how the diet works in great detail later, but for now here are some key points about the diet:

- It is based on sound scientific research and has been scientifically proven.

- It provides all the nutrients you need to stay healthy.

- It can help you stay symptom-free in the long term – some people have stayed on the diet and lived symptom-free for months and even years.

- It won't cure your IBS, but it will help to prevent triggering your symptoms.

If you have been troubled by IBS in the past, we feel confident that you will find great relief in following the Low-FODMAP Diet outlined in this book. Once you're up and running, you might need to keep referring to the book as you go, but with time the diet will become second nature to you. Soon you'll simply feel better than you ever did, without having to put too much effort into how. And using the recipes in this book will help make your process of adaptation to the diet much smoother.

We hope to hear of your success stories, so please feel free to write to us via this book's website, foodintolerancemanagementplan.com.au, or our publishers.

Sincere best wishes for good health.

Dr Sue Shepherd   *Dr Peter Gibson*

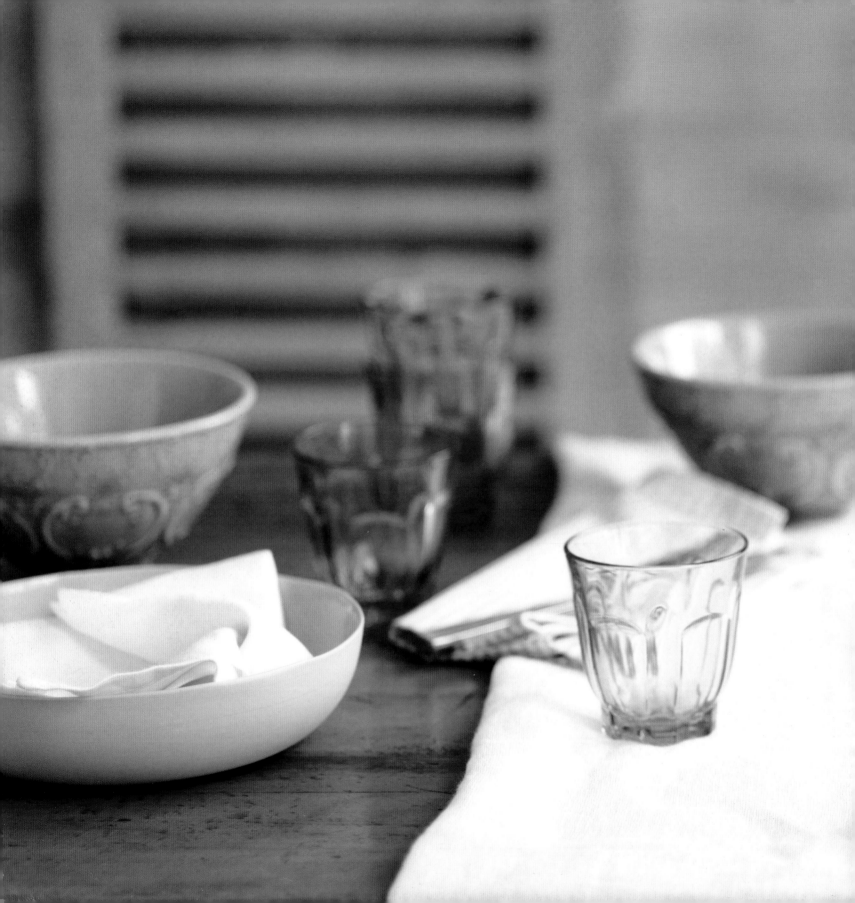

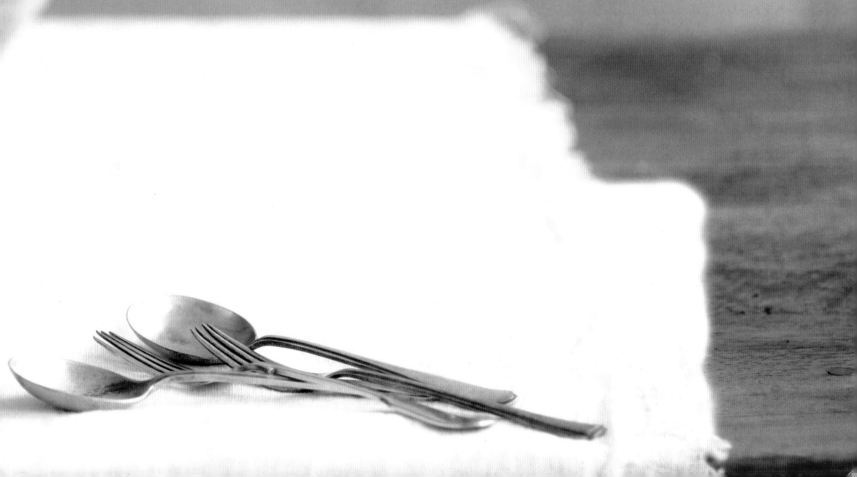

Part One

All about the low-FODMAP diet

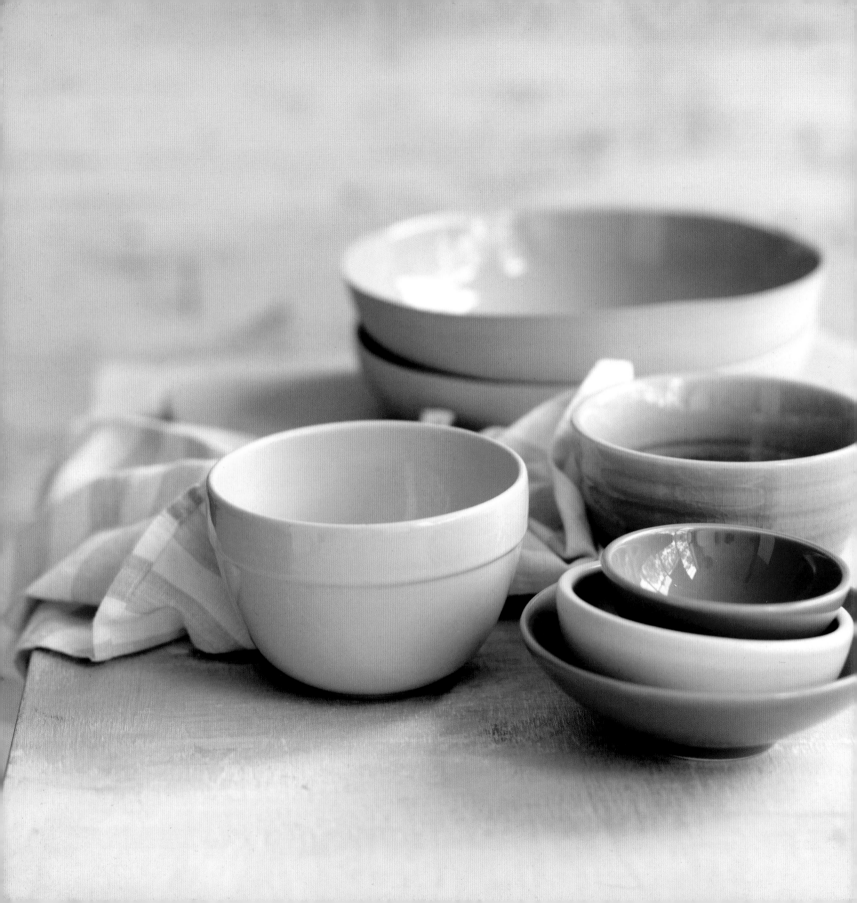

chapter one

How food can trigger gut symptoms

THE TERMS 'food allergy', 'food hypersensitivity' and 'food intolerance' are often used interchangeably and quite incorrectly. There are two very different types of adverse reaction to food:

1. *immunological reactions*. These are reactions to a protein in the food and involve the immune system. This type of reaction, often called a *food allergy* or *food hypersensitivity*, is quite uncommon (affecting about one in 50 people). These reactions are always reproducible, reliable responses to particular foods that occur even with a small amount of the food.

2. *non-immunological reactions*. These reactions do not involve the immune system and are usually referred to as *food intolerances*. They are very common (affecting about one in five people). These reactions can vary and depend on the amount consumed, timing of the meal, and other meals consumed in that day.

Food allergies and food hypersensitivities

These are immune reactions to a specific component in a food (called an allergen), which is almost always a protein. Symptoms include hives, asthma, a runny nose and mouth-swelling. The foods that most commonly cause allergies are: shellfish, eggs, fish, milk, tree-nuts, peanuts, sesame seeds, soy, and wheat, rye, oats and barley. With food allergies, the body reacts to the allergen by producing an antibody to it or with other immune responses. The symptoms experienced depend on the immunological reaction within the body.

FOOD ALLERGIES

In a true food allergy, the body makes antibodies known as immunoglobulin E (IgE). When the antibodies and the allergen meet, they trigger the release of histamine and other defensive chemicals into the body. These chemicals can cause reactions in the mouth, gut, skin, lungs, and heart and blood vessels. Symptoms can include itching, burning and swelling of the mouth, a runny nose, a skin rash, diarrhoea and abdominal cramps, breathing difficulties, vomiting and nausea. In severe cases they can be life-threatening – a reaction called anaphylaxis, in which the circulatory system collapses. People with food allergies may experience gut symptoms, but they are usually minor compared with their other symptoms.

FOOD HYPERSENSITIVITY

Immune responses that do not involve IgE antibodies are often referred to as *food hypersensitivities*. The symptoms related to food hypersensitivity may only affect the gut. These reactions are not easy to diagnose because they don't usually produce antibodies that can be detected in a blood test. One way to help determine whether certain food proteins are causing specific immune responses is to inject them under the skin and look for reactions. But unfortunately these tests don't tell us what is causing the gut symptoms, because the response to proteins in the gut is often very different from that under the skin. The current method of detecting food hypersensitivities is to place the patient on a bland elimination diet, and then, if their symptoms improve, challenging with specific food components. This can be a very long process.

This book and the Low-FODMAP Diet are not designed for people with food allergies or hypersensitivity. If you think you might have a food allergy or hypersensitivity, contact the allergy centres of major hospitals or the Australasian Society of Clinical Immunology and Allergy (ASCIA).

COELIAC DISEASE

WHAT IS IT?

Coeliac disease is an extreme example of food hypersensitivity. It is the result of an immune reaction to gluten that severely injures the body, and has been called an auto-immune disease (because the body turns on itself). Gluten is the main protein in wheat, rye, barley and oats. When someone with coeliac disease eats foods containing gluten, the lining of their bowel is damaged by the white blood cells of their immune system (not by antibodies as in a food allergy).

SYMPTOMS

These range from none at all to nausea, wind, bloating, altered bowel habits (constipation or diarrhoea or a combination of both), fatigue of varying severity, and even skin rashes and liver or neurological problems. It can cause vitamin and mineral deficiencies (particularly of iron, folic acid, zinc and vitamin D) and can also cause malnutrition through weight-loss and loss of muscle mass (although this is less common these days).

TREATMENT

The only way to treat coeliac disease is with a gluten-free diet for life: no wheat, rye, barley or oats, and no products derived from them, ever. It usually requires a major change in diet, but as a rule the gut symptoms, fatigue and other problems disappear over time and the bowel slowly heals. Many complications can occur if coeliac disease is not recognised and treated, including thinning of the bones, infertility, miscarriage, liver disease and even lymphoma, a cancer of the lymph glands. This is why it is so important to investigate the cause of gut symptoms. About one in 20 people with irritable bowel syndrome have coeliac disease.

DIAGNOSIS

The diagnosis of coeliac disease is through blood tests to measure certain types of antibodies that occur only in people with coeliac disease. If blood tests are positive then a gastroscopy (an examination of the upper gut using an endoscope) is performed and tissue samples are taken from the duodenum (the beginning of the small bowel). The samples are examined to see if the bowel lining is damaged in the pattern typical of coeliac disease.

Before the tests, patients are asked to consume foods that contain gluten (e.g. four slices of bread per day) for six weeks. If the tests are negative (normal) but you have been following a gluten-free diet, neither you nor your doctor will be any the wiser about whether you have coeliac disease, and you will need to undergo the tests again. It is *essential* to have these tests before you start trying a gluten-free diet.

THE HUMAN GUT

The gut is also known as the gastrointestinal tract, the digestive tract and the alimentary tract. The main job of the gut is to take in food, break it down so that energy and nutrients can be extracted, and then expel the remaining waste.

It is easiest to think of the gut as a tube that runs from the mouth to the anus. This 8-metre-long tube is made up of many parts, each of which performs a specialised function. After you swallow your food, it enters the *oesophagus*, which pushes the food down into your *stomach*, where food is liquefied and sterilised, and digestion begins. The semi-digested food then passes into the *small intestine* or *small bowel*. The small intestine has three sections with different roles in breaking down food and absorbing nutrients: the *duodenum*, the *ileum* and the *jejunum*.

The leftovers then move into the *large intestine* or *large bowel*, where salts and water are reabsorbed as the contents pass slowly around the several components of the large bowel: the *caecum*, the *ascending colon*, the *transverse colon*, the *descending colon* and the *rectum*. The contents are packaged into stools which are then excreted via the *anus*.

While some *intestinal bacteria* are present in the small bowel, the large bowel contains vast numbers of them. These bacteria feast on undigested or indigestible food, producing short-chain fatty acids that nourish the lining of the large bowel, and gas that contributes to wind.

The whole process of mixing and movement of contents around the gut is controlled by a complex of nerves in the wall of the gut, known as the *enteric nervous system* (ENS) or 'gut brain'. For more on the human gut and the ENS, see the comprehensive information on this book's website, foodintolerancemanagementplan.com.au.

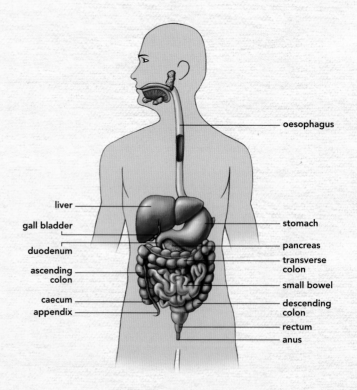

oesophagus

liver

gall bladder

duodenum

ascending colon

caecum
appendix

stomach

pancreas

transverse colon

small bowel

descending colon

rectum

anus

Food intolerances

Unlike food allergy and hypersensitivity, *food intolerance* does not involve the immune system. Food intolerances are the most common trigger of gut symptoms, but can also cause other symptoms, such as headaches and fatigue. This book and the Low-FODMAP Diet are designed to help sufferers of food intolerances. There are two main ways that food intolerances can manifest themselves in gut symptoms:

1. By inducing bowel distension, and thus triggering gut symptoms. This is by far the most common way by which symptoms occur, and the FODMAP sugars (see Chapter 3) are common triggers.

2. By specific responses to foods containing high levels of bioactive substances and food chemicals that either occur naturally in foods or are added during food processing. Common examples include: caffeine, salicylates, amines, glutamate, and colourings and preservatives. Please refer to the ASCIA website for further information.

Irritable bowel syndrome

Irritable bowel syndrome (IBS) is one of a group of conditions called 'functional gastrointestinal disorders'. This means that they cause disturbances in the *function* of the gut but don't have any identifiable physical features, such as ulcers, inflammation, thickening of tissues, lumps and bumps or abnormal blood tests, all of which would indicate a different condition. The diagnosis of IBS relies upon the types of symptoms experienced and their context, such as how long they have been experienced and when they occur.

Functional gastrointestinal disorders are the most common gut conditions – they affect about one in five people. While doctors are good at diagnosing IBS, they don't have much of a track record in fixing the problem. An abundance of 'cures' may well be touted in books and on the internet, but few of them have any scientific basis or have been proven to be effective. Our Low-FODMAP Diet, however, has been scientifically proven to relieve the symptoms of IBS.

Most people with *food allergies* do not have IBS. *Food hypersensitivity* can be an underlying problem in some people who have IBS, but the symptoms of IBS are most commonly triggered by a *food intolerance*. If you suffer from IBS, you very likely have a food intolerance – this book is for you.

THE SYMPTOMS OF IBS

Sufferers of IBS can experience a broad range of symptoms, including abdominal pain and discomfort, bloating, changes in bowel habits, heartburn, nausea, overfullness, and so on. Some of these symptoms originate in the upper gut (the oesophagus and stomach) while others originate in the bowel. Other symptoms or perceived symptoms can include excessive wind, unsatisfied defaecation (incomplete emptying), passage of slimy mucus into the toilet bowl, a noisy abdomen (the noises are called borborygmi) and pain in the rectum. Tiredness is also common and its severity usually depends on that of the bowel symptoms. Muscle aches and pains (called fibromyalgia) occur in some people, while others experience an 'irritable bladder' (urinary frequency and urgency).

DEFINITION AND DIAGNOSIS OF IBS

The official medical definition of IBS is part of what is called the 'Rome III' classification. It says that people can be diagnosed as having IBS if they say they have suffered symptoms of a functional gut disorder for at least six months and have experienced for at least three months of the year mid- or lower abdominal pain or discomfort associated with abdominal bloating or distension, along with changes in bowel habits (diarrhoea, constipation or both). The sufferer need not have experienced all these symptoms and they need not have occurred together, but they often do. The time limits are used to differentiate IBS from acute, one-off tummy upsets that everyone has from time to time.

A typical diagnostic process is as follows:

1. *Identification of symptoms suggestive of IBS*. Your doctor will look for the 'ABC' of IBS – **a**bdominal pain or discomfort, **b**loating and **c**hanges in bowel habits.

2. *Identification of other symptoms*. Your doctor will try to identify 'alarm symptoms' or 'red flags' that may indicate another condition rather than IBS. For example, if the symptoms started after age 50, or if there is blood in the stools, fever, weight-loss of more than 5 kilograms, symptoms that wake you up at night, or a strong family history of bowel cancer, then your doctor will investigate the possibility of inflammatory bowel disease, cancer or other causes, depending upon the situation.

3. *Examination for signs of illness*. IBS is seldom associated with any physical indications of illness.

4. *Provisional diagnosis of IBS*.

5. *Further investigation*. This should always include a blood test for coeliac disease, and, in some people, extra blood tests with or without an endoscopic examination of the stomach and duodenum (called a gastroscopy) and of the colon (called a colonoscopy).

6. *Definitive diagnosis of IBS*. If the tests reveal no other potential cause for the symptoms, then you will be diagnosed with IBS.

Once the diagnosis is complete, you and your doctor will start working on treatment for your IBS. One of the best ways we know of treating the symptoms of IBS is by following the Low-FODMAP Diet, which has been proven to relieve symptoms in three-quarters of IBS sufferers. For more about how to incorporate the Low-FODMAP Diet into your life, read on.

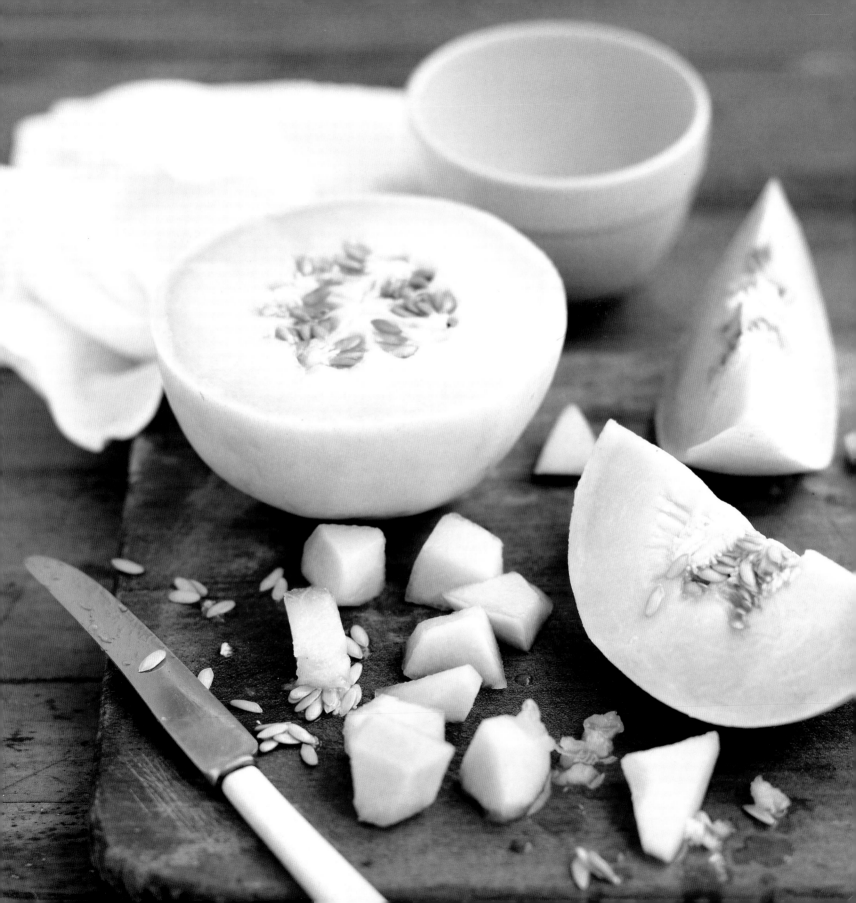

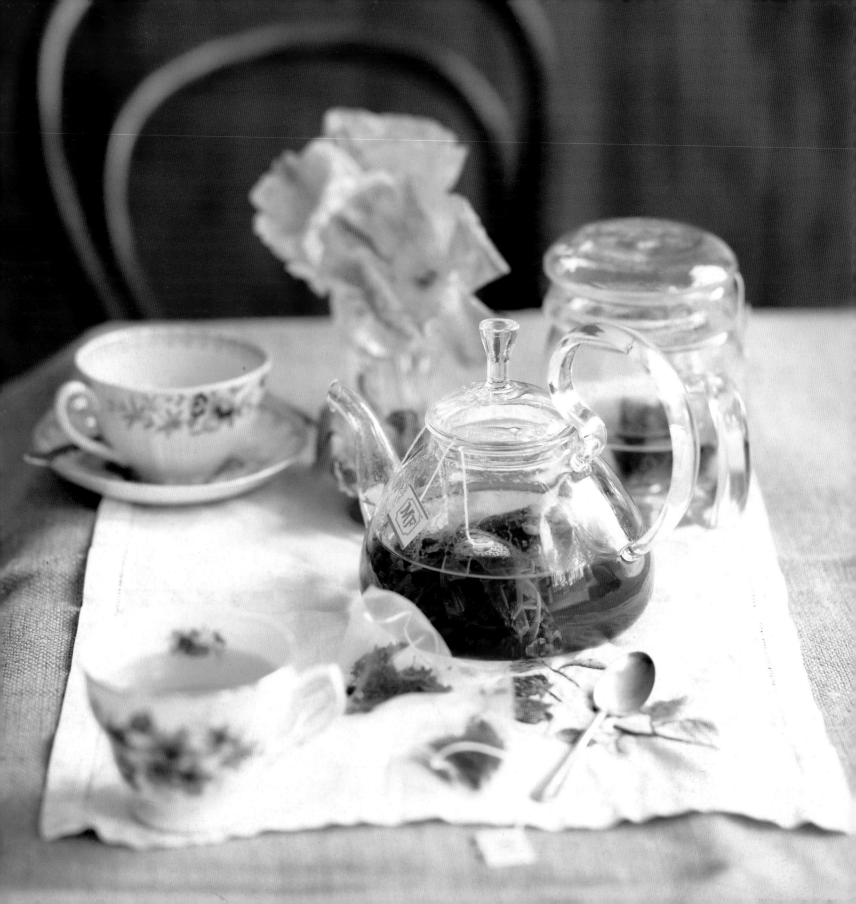

chapter two
What is IBS?

What causes IBS?

We really don't know why some people get IBS and others do not, but one day a single cause might be recognised and a cure found. As far as we can tell, there is no simple infection or other cause that brings about IBS. What we *do* know is that the 'tuning' of the complex nervous system that controls the gut, called the enteric nervous system (ENS), is involved. When the ENS is badly tuned, the result can be an extra-sensitive nerve response in the gut (called visceral hypersensitivity) and/or abnormalities in how the gut moves and deals with its contents. But what actually puts the ENS out of tune and what keeps it out of tune is largely a mystery.

It seems that many factors can contribute to the development of IBS, including:

1. *Genetic factors*. We know from studies of twins that genes play at least some role in IBS, and it is not unusual for IBS to occur within a family.

2. *Gut infections*. For example, when large communities have been infected by a water-borne germ that causes severe diarrhoea, many people have later developed IBS (with diarrhoea as the main symptom). This is called *post-infectious IBS*, and people who suffer from it may have an ongoing very mild inflammation of the gut. Unfortunately, anti-inflammatory drugs seem to have no benefit.

3. *Stress and other psychological factors*. These can affect the ENS by altering how the nerve signals from the gut are transmitted to and interpreted by the brain and spinal cord. The links between the brain and the ENS are collectively called the 'brain–gut axis'. Disturbances in this axis can contribute to IBS and affect anyone.

4. *Abnormal balance of bowel bacteria*. Disturbances in the balance of the bacteria that live in the large bowel may contribute to IBS. This is called *dysbiosis*, and there are different theories about how it might affect the bowel or why it occurs:

- *small intestinal bacterial overgrowth* – one new and quite controversial theory is that IBS is caused by the growth of too many bacteria in the small bowel.

- *food-related causes* – what we eat influences the relative number of different types of bacteria in our bowel. Whether these changes can actually cause IBS symptoms by changing the way the ENS is tuned is the subject of ongoing research.

- *early childhood exposure* – we develop our own set of bacterial types in our bowel at an early age, and it is possible that in some people an interaction between these bacteria and their exposure to aspects of the environment (not just food) dictates how their ENS is tuned.

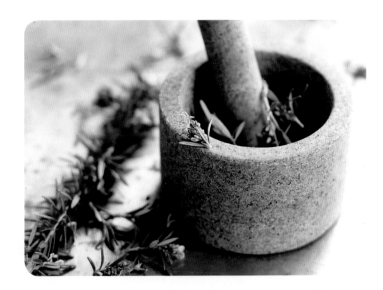

What causes the symptoms of IBS?

Here are a few facts about the origin of the most common symptoms of IBS: bloating and distension; abdominal pain and discomfort; changes in bowel habits; variations in the characteristics of stools; excessive wind; a noisy abdomen; and fatigue.

BLOATING AND DISTENSION

Bloating is defined as the *feeling* of increased pressure in the abdomen, whereas distension is a *measurable* change in the circumference of the abdomen. Distension typically increases for IBS sufferers during the day and after eating. Distension and bloating can be experienced simultaneously or separately. By far the majority of bloating and distension appears to originate in the bowel.

There are only three things that can distend the bowel – solids, liquids or gases. Excesses of these in the bowel cause bloating and distension because they increase the size of the bowel, causing it to take up much more space within the abdomen.

Solids

The only place where any solid matter is retained is the large bowel. Excessive amounts of solid, as may occur in constipation, can cause distension. The large bowel is built to accommodate a fairly large capacity and so it handles distension better than the small bowel. The best way to determine whether the large bowel is overfull is by X-raying the abdomen. And the best way to determine whether this is contributing to the feeling of bloating is to clear the bowel out (under medical supervision) and seeing if this relieves the bloating.

Liquids and gases

Excessive amounts of liquid and gas in the bowel, particularly the last metre of the small bowel and the first parts of the large bowel, are the most common cause of distension, particularly when the distension and bloating vary in severity during the day. How much liquid is retained in the bowel and how much gas is produced depend largely on what food is eaten.

During the digestion process, water and salts are drawn into the body through the walls of the small and large bowel (a process called absorption). If this process is disturbed by illnesses such as a gut infection, pancreatic disease, coeliac disease or inflammatory bowel disease, more liquid will remain in the bowel, which is why diarrhoea is often caused by these conditions.

One way our body maintains its balance is to ensure that the total number of molecules in bodily fluids per unit volume (e.g. per millilitre) remains constant. If you ingest a lot of molecules that cannot be absorbed from the bowel into the bloodstream, the only way your body can keep the number of molecules per unit volume the same is to increase the amount of water retained in your bowel. The bowel usually responds to all this extra fluid by increasing the speed at which it propels the contents, which may lead to diarrhoea. Our diet typically includes many foods containing sugars that are poorly absorbed in the small bowel. All these sugars in the bowel result in more water being retained there. We have called such sugars FODMAPs (see page 23) and our diet for IBS sufferers is based on avoidance of these sugars.

Gas is produced by intestinal bacteria as they feed on unabsorbed food molecules that reach the large bowel. The process by which they do this is called fermentation, and many of us know from making bread or beer that fermentation generates lots of gas. When bacteria ferment carbohydrates (such as sugars), the gases produced are mostly hydrogen and carbon dioxide, although many also produce methane. These odourless gases are produced in large amounts. A small amount of carbon dioxide will travel down the remaining part of the gut and be expelled as wind, but most of the carbon dioxide produced is either used by bacteria for other purposes or absorbed into the bloodstream across the lining of the large bowel, taken up to the lungs and breathed out. Likewise, some of the hydrogen is incorporated by the bacteria into short-chain fatty acids, converted (with carbon dioxide) into methane, or used to make hydrogen sulphide. The rest will be absorbed into the bloodstream and breathed out in the lungs.

FODMAPs

Many carbohydrates in food are poorly digested and are not absorbed by the small bowel. Dietary fibre is one example. Some fibre, known as insoluble fibre, cannot be fermented by bacteria, and other fibre, known as soluble fibre, can be fermented by bacteria. Some sugars, oligosaccharides (short chains of sugars) and sugar alcohols are also indigestible and/or cannot be absorbed by the bowel, but can be broken down by intestinal bacteria to produce gas.

Low Carb diet

One way to reduce the amount of gas in the bowel is to eat a minimal amount of carbohydrates, except for those that are readily digested, such as sucrose (cane sugar) or glucose – although we do not recommend eating lots of these foods. A much better and more practical approach is to determine which carbohydrates are the major contributors to the production of gas in the bowel and to avoid them. These are the carbohydrates that are easily and rapidly fermented by bacteria (they could be considered bacterial 'fast food') – the molecules we call FODMAPs. We know from our scientific studies that FODMAPs can cause diarrhoea, gas production and excess wind. We have also found that the Low-FODMAP Diet reduces bloating, distension and wind in most people.

ABDOMINAL PAIN AND DISCOMFORT

The major cause of abdominal pain and discomfort in IBS is distension of the bowel. How much pain and discomfort is experienced depends on the sensitivity of the nerve endings in the bowel. If they are very sensitive, we say the person has *visceral hypersensitivity*.

We can determine whether someone has visceral hypersensitivity by doing what we call barostat studies. One way is to insert a tube with an attached inflatable balloon into the rectum via the anus. In people without IBS, we can inflate the balloon quite a bit before they experience pain or discomfort, but most people with IBS will experience pain with much less inflation of the balloon. These experiments show that people with IBS require less distension before their nerves send messages to their brain to indicate that they are in pain. In other words, people with IBS appear to have more sensitive nerve endings that react earlier to small amounts of stimulation, so that they experience pain when someone without IBS would not. Another cause of abdominal discomfort is severe contraction of the muscles in the gut wall, causing cramping abdominal pain.

The important feature of bowel pain is that we feel it over a large area of the lower, middle or upper abdomen, but can seldom say exactly where it's coming from. Unlike the skin, where there are lots of pain receptors so that our conscious brain knows exactly where the source of pain is, the abdomen has only general pain receptors, which means that our conscious brain can only recognise that something is happening inside a large part of the abdomen. Usually (but not always), pain from the stomach and duodenum is felt in the upper abdomen, from the small bowel in the middle abdomen, and from the large bowel in the lower abdomen.

WHY DON'T WE ALL SUFFER FROM IBS?

We all eat FODMAPs and produce gas, so why do only some people get IBS? There are five possible reasons:

1. *How much gas we make.* This depends upon the types of bacteria living in our bowel and how they dispose of the gas. Everyone's bowel has a different combination of bacteria, and some bacteria are vigorous fermenters while others produce less gas.

2. *The visceral sensitivity of our bowel.* This is more pronounced in some people. The sensation of bloating depends upon how our ENS is 'tuned' (see page 12) and what degree of distension occurs before we experience discomfort.

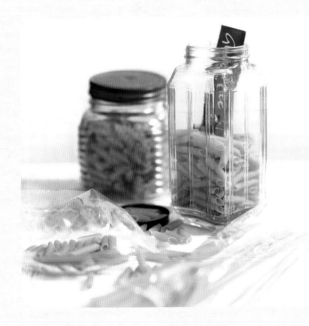

3. *How well our abdominal wall can move gas once it is formed.* Usually, when a lot of gas is introduced into the bowel, this stimulates the digestive tract to move the gas rapidly down the bowel until it is expelled as wind. In some people with IBS, however, the gas just sits around in the bowel, causing more distension.

4. *How well our bowel reacts to distension.* Usually, when the bowel is distended, our stomach muscles tighten automatically, without any input from the brain, so that our abdomen does not stick out. In some people with IBS, however, these reflex responses are very weak. When the bowel is distended, the diaphragm (a large muscle that sits below the lungs) usually becomes more relaxed, allowing more space for the bowel in the abdomen. In some people with IBS, however, bowel distension can lead to contraction and therefore flattening of the diaphragm, which causes more obvious distension and greater discomfort.

5. *Our awareness of signals from the gut and how we interpret them.* We interpret signals from the gut differently under different circumstances. Our perceptions do change according to our levels of stress and anxiety, and according to what is going on in our life. This is also part of the 'brain–gut axis' in action.

CHANGES IN BOWEL HABITS

The nature of our bowel actions – loose as in diarrhoea or hard and dry as in constipation – depends largely on their water content.

Diarrhoea means that the amount of liquid in the bowel has exceeded the ability of the bowel to dry out its contents. There can be three main reasons for this:

1. The amount of liquid coming from the small bowel is too great.

2. The drying-out mechanism is impaired (e.g. when the colon is inflamed).

3. The speed at which the contents are travelling through the bowel is too fast for drying-out to occur (the ENS is driving the muscles too vigorously).

Likewise, constipation can be due to:

1. Too little liquid entering the bowel.

2. Drying-out being too efficient because the bowel contents are moving too slowly or bowel-emptying is too poorly coordinated.

3. Not emptying the bowel as soon as the urge occurs.

The amount of water we drink has some influence here: if we do not drink enough, we absorb more salts and water from the bowel and the chance of constipation increases. But we cannot readily increase the amount of water in the large bowel simply by drinking more water, since this water will be absorbed higher up and the excess will be passed in the urine. In other words, if you are constipated, you should make sure you do not get dehydrated, but drinking several litres of water per day will not give any additional benefit.

Transit time

The time it takes for the bowel contents to move from the beginning to the end of the large bowel is called the *transit time*. One factor affecting transit time is the inherent way the ENS is tuned. In some people, transit time will be long, and their normal bowel pattern will be, for example, five times a week with fairly firm stools. Others have a shorter transit time, normally going two to three times a day and producing softer stools.

From this baseline, other factors can change the transit time. One is the nature of the diet. If it contains little fibre, things will move sluggishly along the bowel and constipation might result. In such situations, a switch to a high-fibre diet or taking fibre supplements would work very well. If, on the other hand, the diet contains a large amount of poorly absorbed sugars (FODMAPs), the ENS may respond by directing the colon muscles to expel the bowel contents and the transit time will then become very short.

It is worth noting that narcotics such as codeine can be particularly constipating because they slow the bowel down and so increase the transit time. So if you experience abdominal pain due to IBS, narcotics are not a good option.

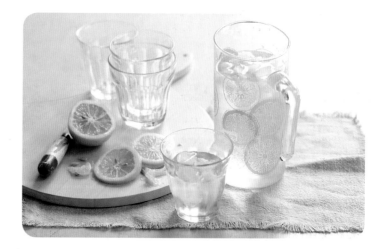

VARIATIONS IN THE CHARACTERISTICS OF STOOLS

People with IBS often query the features of their stools. These can include:

- *Colour* – the colour of the stools does vary, but these variations are not usually significant in IBS.

- *Shape* – ribbon-like or stringy stools, usually associated with straining, indicate constipation. Pellets like sheep droppings also indicate constipation. Floating stools can indicate a good fibre intake.

- *Bits and pieces within the stool* – sometimes people notice tomato skins, corn kernels or seeds in their stools and think this indicates a problem with their digestion, but this is usually only because they have never looked closely before. Many people's stools look like this.

- *Mucus* – it is normal to pass mucus, the slimy stuff that coats the bowel wall, with your stools, and it usually has no serious implications.

- *Blood* – Any blood in the stool warrants a visit to the doctor. It is not part of IBS.

EXCESSIVE WIND

Farting is normal: healthy women fart on average seven times a day and healthy men fourteen times a day. We can expel as much as 2 litres of gas a day; up to half of this might be swallowed air, but the rest is produced in the colon through bacterial fermentation.

There are generally two complaints made about farts:

1. *Frequency*. The way to reduce the volume of gas expelled is to reduce the supply of carbohydrates to the bacteria, by avoiding gas-producing foods rich in FODMAPs, soluble fibre and resistant starch (indigestible starch), and by ensuring that the transit time is not too long.

2. *Smell*. Smelly gas originates from bacterial fermentation of proteins and is produced when the amount of protein ingested exceeds the body's capacity to digest it. This is either because too much protein is being eaten or some of the proteins slip past our digestive mechanisms. Smelly gas usually does not reflect illness or a bad diet.

It is important for bowel health to pass wind when the urge occurs. If you repeatedly ignore the call to pass wind, you may experience abdominal pain and bloating as the wind moves up and down your distended large bowel. If you need to fart, it's better for the sake of your abdomen and wellbeing to move to a place where you can do so with freedom.

NOISY ABDOMEN (BORBORYGMI)

Audible noises and rumblings from the abdomen are called *borborygmi*. These normal events, which may be associated with movement of gas, are a good sign.

FATIGUE

Many people with IBS suffer from fatigue, particularly when their IBS symptoms are bad. The cause of this is usually not known, although there are many theories. The way to deal with fatigue associated with IBS is to reduce the gut symptoms by altering the diet. In some cases, however, the fatigue continues.

Treatment of IBS

Apart from ensuring a good relationship with your doctor (change doctors if you don't think you're getting the attention you need), there are three common modes of treatment for IBS – diet, drugs and psychological therapies – as well as some other, less common therapies.

DIET

People with IBS often know that certain foods will trigger their symptoms and really want to know what they should or should not eat. It has been shown that dietary change is the major way in which sufferers of IBS attempt to help themselves. Unfortunately, until recently doctors tended to shy away from offering specific dietary advice, although they worked hard to eliminate poor eating habits (such as stress-filled meals or always eating on the run) and to avoid obvious dietary extremes (such as too many cups of coffee each day or a diet full of fat or devoid of fibre). Until the Low-FODMAP Diet, there was minimal scientific proof that specific dietary changes helped people with IBS.

Dietitians with expertise in gastrointestinal nutrition and many doctors now recommend the Low-FODMAP Diet as a cornerstone of their treatment for people with IBS. The majority of IBS sufferers who have tried the diet have experienced greatly improved symptoms and a markedly reduced need for medication.

Will a gluten-free diet help with IBS?

A gluten-free diet is often recommended as a way of managing the symptoms of IBS. Many people claim that it effectively relieves the symptoms of IBS, and there are plenty of websites promoting gluten-free diets as a cure for everything from IBS to chronic fatigue syndrome and autism. Often these claims are not backed up by any scientific evidence. A gluten-free diet could improve symptoms of IBS not because it removes gluten from the diet but because it removes fructans, a type of FODMAP, from the diet. Scientifically validated evidence is needed before we can start blaming gluten for symptoms of IBS in people who do not have coeliac disease.

DRUGS

Medications are generally not effective in treating IBS overall, and no drug has been shown to relieve all IBS symptoms. Drugs can, however, play a definite role in treating specific, troublesome symptoms of IBS. Your doctor may recommend medications in response to the major symptom that is causing you distress, such as the following:

- *Abdominal cramping pains* – drugs that relieve spasm, such as mebeverine, anticholinergic drugs or peppermint oil, would be the first choice, followed by antidepressant drugs, usually at low doses.

- *Diarrhoea* – drugs that slow the bowel, such as loperamide or diphenoxylate.

- *Constipation* – ensuring adequate fibre intake, either through diet or with a fibre supplement such as sterculia, or the use of laxatives such as Epsom salts or polyethylene glycol preparations.

- *Sleep disturbance* – perhaps a tricyclic antidepressant.

- *Anxiety and stress* – any of the antidepressants.

Antibiotics are sometimes used to treat 'small intestinal bacterial overgrowth', and do help in some cases, but the concept of bacterial overgrowth is very controversial and it is generally not a good idea to take antibiotics over a long period of time.

PSYCHOLOGICAL THERAPIES

Many people with IBS try psychological approaches like yoga and hypnotherapy to deal with issues such as anxiety and stress that may be contributing to their IBS. There is now a body of evidence, however, that these techniques help symptoms of IBS and work just as well or even better for people who are not so stressed. Cognitive behaviour therapy with a trained psychologist or hypnotherapy with a trained hypnotherapist are less accessible, but there is very good evidence that they provide considerable benefit. 'Gut-directed' hypnotherapy has been shown to have lasting benefits for people with IBS. How and why it works is not well understood, but it deserves attention. If you're considering hypnotherapy, check the credentials and training of the hypnotherapist.

OTHER THERAPIES

Some people with IBS claim that the following therapies have helped relieve their symptoms:

- *Probiotics* – these are friendly bacteria with supposed health benefits, usually various strains of *Lactobacillus* or *Bifidobacteria*, used alone or in combination. Many other types of bacteria (and even yeast) have also been marketed as probiotics. These have to be taken every day, as the bacteria do not remain in the gut for long. One good thing about probiotics is that they are unlikely to do any harm (apart from lightening the wallet – they're not cheap!). The problem is that few have actually been proven in clinical trials to be of significant benefit.

- *Prebiotics* – these are carbohydrates, such as inulin (not to be confused with insulin) and fructose-oligosaccharide (also known as FOS or oligofructose), that specifically encourage the growth of 'good' bacteria and reduce the number of supposedly 'bad' bacteria. There is no evidence that these help in IBS, and in fact they are likely to cause *more* IBS symptoms, since they behave like or are FODMAPs. We currently do not recommend them.

- *Exercise* – walking or simple exercises at the gym (rather than running marathons) may be beneficial.

- *Acupuncture* – some people claim that acupuncture relieves their IBS symptoms, particularly abdominal pain. It remains unproven scientifically, but if your acupuncturist is appropriately trained and skilled, it is unlikely to do you any harm.

- *Traditional Chinese medicine* – one Australian study showed this to be effective for IBS, but there are so many variations in the herbs that are used that it is not easy to generalise. If you do try this treatment, find a practitioner with experience in treating IBS.

- *Other treatments* – some sufferers claim that aromatherapy and homeopathy have helped them, but there is no scientific evidence at all that either of these techniques works.

The Low-FODMAP Diet and IBS

The Low-FODMAP Diet has been proven to work in the treatment of IBS symptoms in both the short and long term. Once you know how to follow the diet, it is self-directed and self-empowering, meaning there are no ongoing costs for consultations or drugs. In the next chapter you'll learn all about the Low-FODMAP Diet – how it works and what it involves.

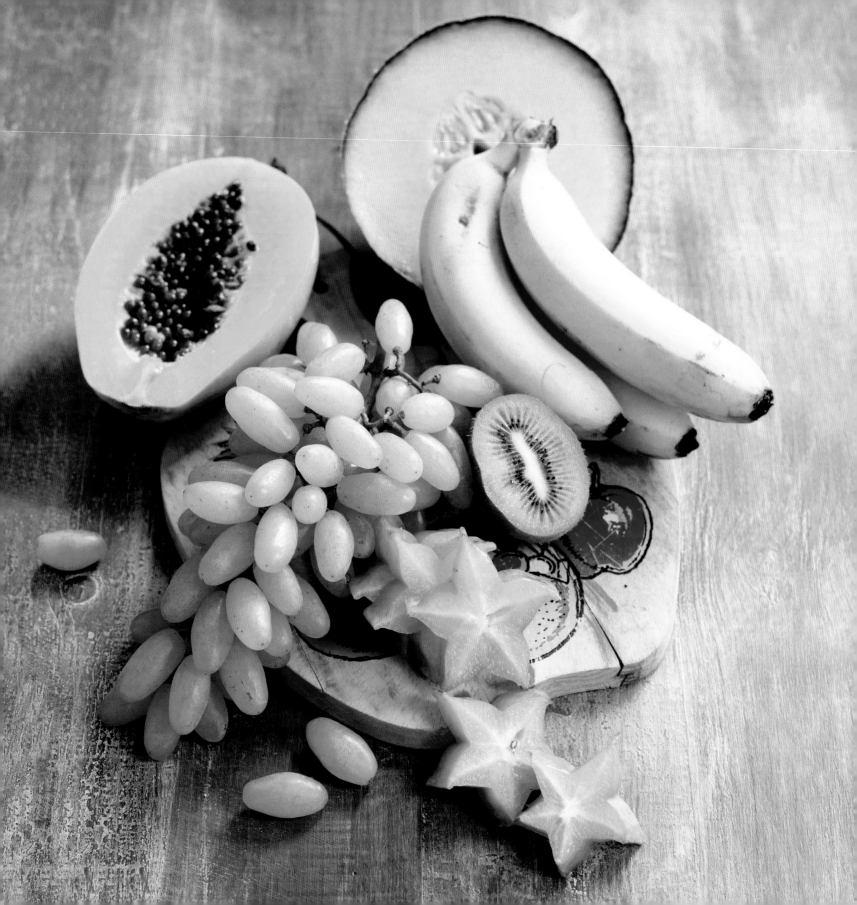

chapter three

All about the Low-FODMAP Diet

WE'VE ALREADY SEEN how the foods we eat can cause the symptoms of irritable bowel syndrome (IBS). Many people who experience IBS have already recognised a strong association between what they eat and the severity of their symptoms.

Many IBS sufferers find the idea of changing their diet much more appealing than taking medication. It means they are taking action themselves to relieve their symptoms, and that feeling of empowerment regarding our own health is important. Others, however, prefer to take medication – because it requires no effort on their part and is a 'quick fix'. Unfortunately, there is no such thing as a 'quick fix'. As we have seen, drugs can relieve *some* symptoms, but they are not very effective overall, they often come with side effects and they can be costly. You are far better off in the long term trying to change your diet.

DIETITIANS

Before you try the Low-FODMAP Diet you may want to consult an Accredited Practising Dietitian who specialises in IBS. The dietitian would look at your patterns of eating, identify the food triggers for your symptoms and ensure that your diet remains nutritionally adequate. If you would like to follow the Low-FODMAP Diet with the help of your dietitian, let them know this before your first visit. For more on this, visit this book's website, foodintolerancemanagementplancom.au.

General eating advice

Apart from following the Low-FODMAP Diet, there are some simple rules you can observe with your food intake that could well help reduce the severity of your IBS symptoms.

MEAL PATTERN AND SIZE

Our eating patterns can by themselves trigger gut symptoms. Here are some tips that could help:

- *Don't overeat, and enjoy your meals while eating slowly*. Overeating or 'binge eating' (devouring large quantities of foods in a short period of time) can increase IBS symptoms. Eating small meals means you will consume smaller amounts of food triggers such as FODMAPs.

- *Avoid excessive intake of fats, caffeine and alcohol*. People with IBS have a lower threshold for bloating, discomfort and pain after high-fat meals, so avoid rich, greasy food. A low to moderate intake of fat, caffeine and alcohol is best both for long-term health and minimising the symptoms of IBS.

- *Avoid stress-filled meals*. Don't use mealtimes as a forum for difficult family discussions or work emails. Take time out to consciously enjoy your meal.

- *Don't skip meals – eat regularly*. People often skip meals as a way to avoid excessive calorie intake, but hunger might encourage rapid overeating at the next meal. Breakfast is an important meal. It enables rehydration after many hours of no fluid intake, and promotes a healthier intake of nutrients. Eating breakfast has also been associated with improved school performance.

SHOULD I EAT MORE FIBRE?

There is little to suggest that fibre in the diet, whether too much or too little, causes IBS. The few well-structured scientific studies of whether increased fibre intake affects IBS symptoms have found overall that fibre neither improves nor worsens IBS symptoms. Some people clearly benefit from altering their fibre intake – if you are constipated and your intake of dietary fibre is very low, then increasing your fibre intake is an effective way to reduce your constipation. In contrast, if you are constipated and are consuming a large amount of fibre, reducing the amount of fibre in the diet can help reduce symptoms such as bloating and discomfort. In most people, the best advice is to ensure an adequate intake of fibre – 25–30 grams per day.

You can obtain dietary fibre from wholegrain foods – such as brown rice, buckwheat, oatmeal, whole cornmeal, quinoa and amaranth – and from products made from these, such as pasta, bread and breakfast cereals. You can also obtain fibre from nuts and seeds, and fruits and vegetables – particularly just under the skin, so try to avoid peeling away the goodness.

What are FODMAPS?

We have seen that food intolerances can lead to IBS symptoms. Certain food components cause the bowel to distend by drawing in more fluid and rapidly generating gas when they are fermented by bowel bacteria.

The main dietary components that do this are known as fermentable, poorly absorbed short-chain carbohydrates. In other words, they are indigestible sugars that provide fast food for bowel bacteria. Such sugars have been given the acronym FODMAP which stands for:

Fermentable – rapidly broken down by bacteria in the bowel
Oligosaccharides – fructans and galacto-oligosaccharides (GOS)
Disaccharides – lactose
Monosaccharides – fructose
And
Polyols – sorbitol, mannitol, xylitol and maltitol

If this seems too wordy to get your head around, just remember that 'saccharide' is simply another word for sugar. A monosaccharide has one sugar, a disaccharide has two, an oligosaccharide has only a few (less than ten), and a polysaccharide has a large number (more than ten). Polyols are what we call sugar alcohols, sugar molecules with an alcohol side-chain. You don't need to know anything more than this. You may have heard of some of these sugars or seen them in ingredients lists.

HOW DO WE KNOW THE LOW-FODMAP DIET WORKS?

Our first task was to design the Low-FODMAP Diet. This had never been done before and it was quite a challenge finding information about the FODMAP content of foods. Once we had found this we were able to design the first version of the diet. Our second task was to see if people could understand and follow the diet and whether it improved symptoms in people with IBS.

We sought a group of IBS sufferers and taught them how to follow the diet. Four out of five found the diet easy to stick to for a long period of time (months and years) and three out of four found that all of their IBS symptoms (pain, bloating and change in bowel habits) improved markedly. This improvement was greater than we had seen for any drug or other treatment approach. This was only a preliminary experiment, however. We still needed to prove that the results were not due to the 'placebo effect'.

To do this, we rechallenged the patients whose symptoms improved on the Low-FODMAP Diet, this time with a double-blind, quadruple-arm, randomised, cross-over placebo-controlled rechallenge trial in twenty-five people. This means that we tested twenty-five people by putting them on or off the diet, without them or us knowing whether or not they were taking in FODMAPs.

We supplied these twenty-five people, all of whom had fructose malabsorption, with all their food, which contained no FODMAPs, for twenty-two weeks. In four separate periods of two weeks at a time, the participants added a drink to all of their meals. This drink contained fructans alone, fructose alone, fructans *and* fructose together, or glucose alone (this was the dummy or placebo – most people should absorb glucose without any problems). The drinks all tasted the same, and neither we nor the participants knew which one they were taking. We asked all participants to score the severity of their symptoms every day during the study.

At the end of the study, all the data were locked so that we could make no changes, and then which participant had which drink was revealed to us. Our analysis of the results showed that, during those dietary periods when FODMAPs were taken, the participants experienced markedly more symptoms than when only glucose was taken. The fructose alone and fructans alone had similar effects (proving to the sceptics that it is not only fructose that is important) and the fructose and fructans had additive effects (i.e. the symptoms were more pronounced when the two sugars were consumed together).

These results have now been published in a high-ranking peer-reviewed international medical journal. The FODMAP concept has been proven.

We also showed that the diet works for the majority of people with IBS symptoms who do not have fructose malabsorption, and in people with IBS symptoms and inflammatory bowel disease (ulcerative colitis and Crohn's disease, see page 56).

We have since looked further into the FODMAP content of various foods and have used this information to refine the Low-FODMAP Diet. This work is ongoing and we will add our findings to this book's website, foodintolerancemanagementplan.com.au, as they become available.

How do FODMAPS cause symptoms of IBS?

FODMAPs all have the same characteristics:

1. *They are poorly absorbed in the small bowel*. This means that many of these molecules arrive from the stomach into the small bowel but don't get absorbed, instead passing right through to the colon. This occurs either because they cannot be broken down or they are slow to be absorbed. We all differ in our ability to digest and absorb some FODMAPs – fructose absorption is slow in all of us but very slow in some, some people do not make enough enzyme to break down lactose, and the ability to absorb polyols, which are the wrong shape to pass readily through the lining of the small bowel, varies from person to person. Since none of us can digest fructans and galacto-oligosaccharides (GOS), they are poorly absorbed in everyone.

2. *They are small molecules, consumed in a concentrated dose*. When small, concentrated molecules are poorly absorbed, the body tries to 'dilute' them by forcing water into the gastrointestinal tract. Extra fluid in the gastrointestinal tract can cause diarrhoea and affect the muscular movement of the gut.

3. *They are 'fast food' for the bacteria that live naturally in the large bowel*. The large bowel (and the lower part of the small bowel) naturally contains billions of bacteria. If molecules are not absorbed in the small bowel, they continue the journey to the large bowel. The bacteria that live there see these food molecules as 'fast food' and quickly break them down, which

produces hydrogen, carbon dioxide and methane gases. How quickly the molecules are fermented depends on their chain length – oligosaccharides and sugars are fermented very rapidly compared with fibre, which contains much longer chain molecules, known as polysaccharides.

Multiple types of FODMAPs are usually present in any one meal. Because they all cause distension in the same way once they reach the lower small bowel and colon, their effects are cumulative. This means that the degree of bowel distension can depend upon the total FODMAPs consumed, not just the amount of any individual FODMAP consumed. If someone who cannot digest lactose well and absorbs fructose poorly eats a meal that contains some lactose, some fructans, some polyols, some GOS and some fructose, the effect on the bowel will be 1 + 1 + 1 + 1 + 1 = 5 times greater than if they ate the same amount of only one of those. That is why we have to consider all FODMAPs in food when modifying our diet.

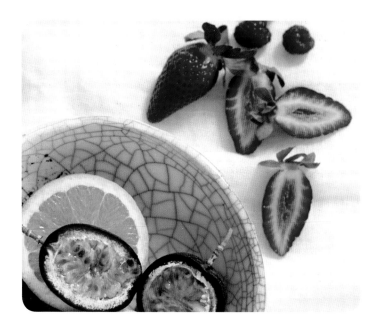

Introducing the FODMAPS

The nature of each type of FODMAP and which foods contain them is outlined below.

OLIGOSACCHARIDES

The major types of oligosaccharides that are FODMAPs are fructans and galacto-oligosaccharides (GOS).

Fructans

Fructans are chains of fructose molecules with a glucose molecule at the end. The main dietary sources of fructans include wheat products (breads, cereals and pasta) and some vegetables, such as onions. Additional sources of fructans are inulins and fructo-oligosaccharide (also called oligofructose and FOS), which are added to some foods, such as some yoghurts and milk, as a prebiotic (see page 19).

No one is able to digest fructans, and if you have IBS you should minimise your intake of them. Fructans are probably the most common FODMAP to cause symptoms of IBS, probably because most people eat a lot of them. They occur in a wide variety of foods and in large amounts in our food supply.

Foods are considered a problem for sufferers of IBS if they contain more than 0.2 grams of fructans per serve of food. The main food sources of fructans are varieties of vegetables and grains, and a small number of fruits.

HIGH-FRUCTAN FOODS	
FRUITS	custard apples, persimmon, rambutan, watermelon
VEGETABLES	artichokes (globe and Jerusalem), asparagus, beetroot, Brussels sprouts, cabbage, chicory, dandelion leaves, fennel, garlic, leeks, okra, onions (brown, red, white, onion powder), peas, radicchio, spring onions (white part)
CEREALS, GRAINS AND STARCHES	*wheat-based products* – bread, pasta, couscous, crackers and biscuits in large amounts *rye-based products* – bread and dry biscuits in large amounts
LEGUMES	chickpeas, lentils, all legume beans
DRINKS	chicory-based coffee-substitutes, dandelion tea
FIBRE SUPPLEMENTS	inulin in some processed foods (e.g. low-fat dairy products) and 'high fibre' or 'fibre enriched' products; fructo-oligosaccharides, often in drinks designed as nutritional supplements

LOW-FRUCTAN ALTERNATIVES

FRUITS	all except custard apples, persimmon, rambutan, watermelon
VEGETABLES	alfalfa, avocados, bamboo shoots, bean shoots, bok choy, broccoli, capsicums (peppers), carrots, cauliflower, celery, chives, choy sum, cucumber, eggplant (aubergine), endive, ginger, green beans, lettuce, marrow, mushrooms, olives, parsnips, potatoes, pumpkin (squash), silverbeet (Swiss chard), snowpeas (mangetout), spinach, spring onions (green part only), squash, swedes, sweet potatoes, taro, tomatoes, turnips, yams, zucchini (courgettes)
CEREALS, GRAINS AND STARCHES	amaranth, arrowroot, barley, buckwheat, corn (maize), millet, oats, potato, quinoa, rice, sorghum, tapioca
DRINKS	regular tea and coffee, herbal teas and infusions
FOOD SUPPLEMENTS	barley bran, chia, LSA (linseed, sunflower, almond mix), nuts and seeds, oat bran, psyllium, rice bran

Galacto-oligosaccharides (GOS)

Galacto-oligosaccharides (GOS) are chain molecules formed from galactose sugars joined together with a fructose and glucose at the end. Raffinose and stachyose are the most common GOS found in food. They occur in legumes, such as baked beans, lentils and chickpeas.

Like fructans, GOS cannot be digested or absorbed by anybody and they should be avoided if you have IBS. High-GOS foods are those that contain more than 0.2 grams per serve.

HIGH-GOS FOODS

LEGUMES	chickpeas, dry beans (e.g. kidney, baked, borlotti, haricot, pinto, navy, lima, butter, adzuki, soy, mung and broad beans), lentils

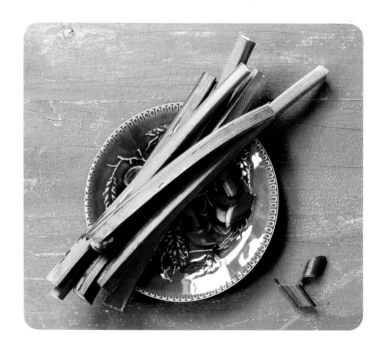

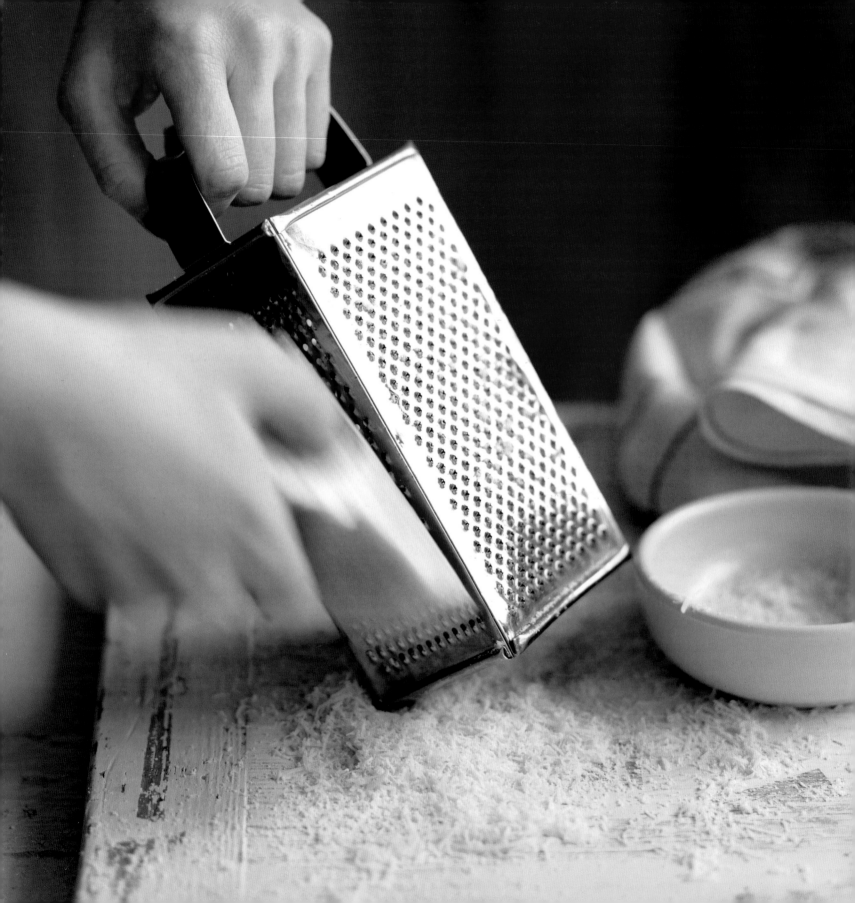

DISACCHARIDES

Only one disaccharide can potentially act as a FODMAP in food – lactose.

Lactose

Lactose is a double sugar that occurs naturally in all animal milks, including milk from cows, sheep and goats. Made up of two digestible sugars called glucose and galactose, it is broken down in the small bowel into its component sugars by an enzyme called lactase. Lactose-intolerant people, however, have low levels of lactase and can therefore only break down a very small amount of the lactose they consume. Such people may benefit from reducing their lactose intake as part of the Low-FODMAP Diet. Experience has shown that reducing lactose intake alone (without also reducing intake of the other FODMAPs) is not very effective in minimising IBS symptoms.

Most people who are lactase-deficient, however, still produce a small amount of the lactase enzyme and do not need to remove lactase completely from their diet.

A lactose-free diet is *not* a dairy-free diet. Lactose is present in varying amounts in milk and milk products such as yoghurt, custards, dairy desserts, ice cream and soft, unripened cheeses (such as cottage, ricotta, quark and cream cheeses). Cream contains a minimal amount of lactose, and hard and ripened cheeses (such as cheddar, tasty, parmesan, camembert, edam, gouda, blue vein and mozzarella) and butter are virtually lactose-free.

Most people with lactose malabsorption can handle up to 4 grams of lactose per serve of food without experiencing problems. A thin spread of margarine and small amounts of milk in tea and coffee, chocolate, cakes and biscuits may be tolerated whereas a full glass of milk would cause symptoms. If you are lactase-deficient you should restrict lactose-containing foods based on your own degree of sensitivity.

LACTOSE CONTENT OF COMMON FOODS AND DRINKS

FOOD OR BEVERAGE (serving size)	LACTOSE (grams)
skim milk (250 ml)	16
evaporated milk (125 ml)	13
low-fat milk (250 ml)	13
full-fat milk (250 ml)	12
low-fat yoghurt (200 g)	9
full-cream yoghurt (200 g)	8
cheesecake (150 g)	6
ice cream (2 scoops)	6
custard (125 ml)	6
milk chocolate (50 g)	5
cream cheese (1 tablespoon)	3
cottage cheese (2 tablespoons)	1
cream (1 tablespoon)	1
sour cream (1 tablespoon)	1
white sauce (2 tablespoons)	1
cake (150 g)	1
butter (20 g)	0.1
cheese – blue vein, bocconcini, brie, cheddar, edam, feta, gouda, mozzarella, Swiss (30 g)	0.1

High-lactose foods contain more than 4 grams of lactose per serve; moderate-lactose foods contain 1–4 grams of lactose per serve; and low-lactose foods contain less than 1 gram per serve. High-lactose foods may be safely consumed in small quantities, as indicated in the following table.

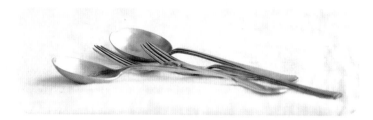

HIGH-LACTOSE FOODS AND ALTERNATIVES

FOOD TYPE	HIGH-LACTOSE FOOD	LOW-LACTOSE ALTERNATIVES
milk	full-fat, low-fat and skim cow's, goat's or sheep's milk	full-fat, low-fat and skim lactose-free milk; soy milk; rice, oat, almond and quinoa milk substitutes (choose calcium-fortified) *small quantities* – small amounts of regular milk in tea and coffee
milk products	custard, ice cream, dairy desserts, milk powder (also called 'milk solids' or 'milk solids non-fat'), evaporated milk, sweetened condensed milk	soy ice cream (choose calcium-fortified) *small quantities* – regular milk or milk powder in cakes, biscuits and snacks (e.g. milk chocolate)
yoghurt	full-fat, low-fat and skim cow's, sheep's and goat's yoghurt, fromage frais	soy yoghurts, lactose-free yoghurts

MODERATE-LACTOSE FOODS AND ALTERNATIVES

FOOD TYPE	MODERATE-LACTOSE FOOD	LOW-LACTOSE ALTERNATIVES
milk product	cream	lactose-free cream
soft cheeses	cottage, cream cheese, creme fraiche, mascarpone, quark, ricotta	small serves of soft cheeses

LOW-LACTOSE FOODS

HARD, FORMED AND RIPENED CHEESES	blue vein, bocconcini, brie, cheddar, colby, edam, emmental, feta, gloucester, gorgonzola, gouda, gruyère, haloumi, havarti, mozzarella, neufchatel, parmesan, pecorino, provolone, raclette, romano, stilton, Swiss, taleggio
BUTTER	all types

MONOSACCHARIDES

The only important monosaccharide that can potentially act as a FODMAP in food is fructose.

Fructose

Fructose, a single sugar, is often referred to as the 'fruit sugar'. It is found in every fruit, in honey, and in high-fructose corn syrup. It is a component of 'sugar' (also called sucrose or cane sugar) and is also found in some vegetables (e.g. sugar snap peas) and grains (e.g. wheat).

When fructose occurs with glucose, it is well absorbed because it is 'piggybacked' across the bowel lining by the glucose. If fructose is found in higher concentrations than glucose, however (a situation we call 'excess fructose'), its absorption is slow or incomplete. This situation is called *fructose malabsorption*. This is not an 'illness' or a 'condition'. It is just a part of a person's physiology – some people are not well equipped to absorb excess fructose while others are. About one in three of us have fructose malabsorption. It is not more common in people with IBS.

If you have fructose malabsorption, there is no need to avoid fructose (or fruit) completely. As long as the fructose is balanced with glucose, or there is more glucose than fructose, you can eat moderate amounts without experiencing IBS symptoms. The following table demonstrates this concept.

CALCULATING THE FREE-FRUCTOSE CONTENT OF FOODS

FOOD	FRUCTOSE (per 100 grams)	GLUCOSE (per 100 grams)	EXCESS FREE FRUCTOSE (column 2 minus column 3)	CONCLUSION
honey	40	30	10	problem
mango	2	1.5	0.5	problem
kiwifruit	**4**	**4**	**0**	**suitable**

Foods are considered a problem for IBS sufferers if they contain more than 0.5 grams fructose in excess of glucose per 100 grams of food. Foods and beverages with 0.1–0.5 grams more fructose than glucose per 100 grams of food do not usually induce symptoms. The main food sources of excess fructose are fruits.

All good things should be enjoyed in moderation. The gut can be overloaded by lots of fructose even if glucose is in balance with the fructose. So you should not only choose fruit in which fructose and glucose are in balance, but also limit the amount of such fruit you eat in one sitting. The total fruit quantity should be approximately equal to the size of an average orange. You can enjoy several serves of fruit per day, but ensure they are spread out, with at least two hours between. An acceptable single fruit intake could be one of the following:

- 1 whole banana or orange.

- 2 kiwifruit or mandarins.

- 1 small slice of melon or pineapple.

- ⅓–½ glass of suitable fruit juice (e.g. orange juice *not* apple or pear juice).

- 1 small handful of berries or grapes.

- A very small amount of suitable dried fruit (e.g. 10 sultanas or an equivalent serving size of banana chips, cranberries, currants, paw paw, pineapple, sultanas or raisins).

- 2 small tomatoes (tomatoes should be treated as a fruit).

- 3 tablespoons tomato paste or suitable fruit-based sauce or chutney.

FOODS CONTAINING EXCESS FREE FRUCTOSE

FRUITS	apples, mangoes, nashi pears, pears, persimmon, rambutan, watermelon
VEGETABLES	sugar snap peas
HONEY	all types
SWEETENERS	high-fructose corn syrup, corn syrup solids, fructose, fruit juice concentrate

LOW-FRUCTOSE OR BALANCED ALTERNATIVES

FRUITS	apricots, avocados, bananas, blackberries, blueberries, boysenberries, cherries, cranberries, cumquats, durian, grapefruit, grapes, honeydew melon, kiwifruit, lemons, limes, longons, lychees, mandarins, nectarines, oranges, passionfruit, paw paw, peaches, pineapple, plums, raspberries, rhubarb, rockmelon (canteloupe), star fruit, strawberries, tangelos, tomatoes
VEGETABLES	all except sugar snap peas
HONEY	golden syrup, maple syrup, molasses, rice syrup, treacle; yeast extracts, peanut butter, choc-nut spreads, jam and marmalade in small quantities (limit intake of '100 per cent fruit spreads', which are often sweetened with pear juice)
SWEETENERS	sucrose (table sugar, cane sugar), including caster sugar, icing sugar, brown sugar, raw sugar; glucose

POLYOLS

Polyols, also called 'sugar alcohols', are given names that end in 'ol' and include sorbitol, mannitol, maltitol and xylitol. Polyols occur naturally in some fruits and vegetables. They are often used in food manufacturing as humectants (water-binding agents) and artificial sweeteners – particularly in 'sugar-free' chewing gums, mints and confectionery. When used as an artificial sweetener, polyols can be identified by their food additive numbers – sorbitol (420), mannitol (421), maltitol (965), xylitol (967). The packaging will state 'Excess consumption may have a laxative effect'. The food additive isomalt (953) may also behave in a similar way. Foods are considered a problem for IBS sufferers if they contain more than 0.5 grams of polyols per serve.

HIGH-POLYOL FOODS

FRUITS	apples, apricots, blackberries, cherries, longons, lychees, nashi pears, nectarines, pears, plums, prunes, watermelon
VEGETABLES	avocados, cauliflower, mushrooms, snowpeas (mange-tout)
'DIET', 'SUGAR-FREE' OR 'LOW-CARB' FOODS	gums, mints, lollies, dairy desserts and other products containing polyol additives (as below); foods with the warning 'Excess consumption may have a laxative effect'
ADDITIVES	sorbitol (420), mannitol (421), maltitol (965), xylitol (967)

LOW-POLYOL ALTERNATIVES

FRUITS	bananas, blueberries, boysenberries, cranberries, durian, grapefruit, grapes, honeydew melon, kiwifruit, lemons, limes, mandarins, mangoes, oranges, passionfruit, paw paw, pineapple, raspberries, rhubarb, rockmelon (canteloupe), star fruit, strawberries, tangelos
VEGETABLES	all except avocados, cauliflower, mushrooms, snowpeas (mange-tout)
'DIET', 'SUGAR-FREE' OR 'LOW-CARB' FOODS	regular chewing gum sweetened with sugar (sucrose), regular sugar-sweetened mints and confectionery
ADDITIVES	aspartame, saccharine, stevia

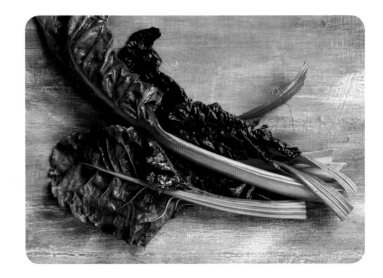

HOW DO WE KNOW WHAT FODMAPS DO IN THE BOWEL?

It is easy to show that the FODMAPs are 'fast food' for bacteria, although we don't suggest you try it at home. Get some faeces, mix it up into a slurry and add any of the FODMAPs. The bacteria in the faeces rapidly ferment the FODMAP added. We know this because as the FODMAP disappears, gas is produced and the slurry becomes more acidic (because acids are produced during fermentation).

We have shown that FODMAPs are poorly absorbed from the small bowel in studies with people who have had an ileostomy (i.e. their large bowel has been removed and the contents of their small bowel empty directly into a bag). Nearly all the FODMAPs consumed in food can be detected in the matter that empties from the ileostomy.

Research by our group at Monash University in people who have had an ileostomy has shown that FODMAPs draw water into the bowel. We fed these people a high-FODMAP diet and then a low-FODMAP diet, or vice versa. The amount of liquid matter that was emptied into the ileostomy bag was much greater when they ate a high-FODMAP diet. This proved that FODMAPs increase the amount of liquid in the bowel. One way to reduce diarrhoea then is to reduce the intake of FODMAPs in the diet.

We can prove that a high-FODMAP diet increases gas production by measuring how much hydrogen is present in the breath of people who have eaten a diet containing the same amount of fibre and starch, but either a lot of or only a few FODMAPs. Hydrogen in the breath comes from gases produced by bacteria in the bowel, and fermentation of carbohydrates by bacteria in the bowel is the only way that hydrogen is produced in the body. We measured the hydrogen in the breath of healthy volunteers and people with IBS. The breath of people in both groups who ate a high-FODMAP diet had increased hydrogen levels compared with those who ate a low-FODMAP diet.

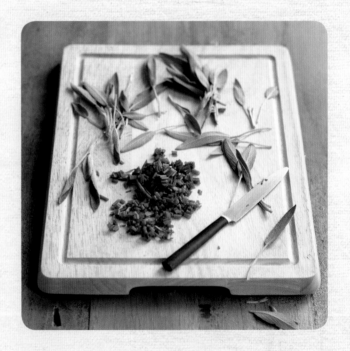

FOODS SUITABLE FOR A LOW-FODMAP DIET

FRUITS _Citrus?_	bananas, blueberries, carambola, durian, grapefruit, grapes, honeydew melon, kiwifruit, lemons, limes, mandarins, oranges, passionfruit, paw paw, raspberries, rockmelon (canteloupe), strawberries, tangelos, tomatoes
VEGETABLES	alfalfa, bamboo shoots, bean shoots, bok choy, broccoli, capsicum (pepper), carrot, celery, choko, choy sum, corn, cucumber, eggplant (aubergine), green beans, lettuce (butter, iceberg), marrow, olives, parsnip, potato, pumpkin (squash), silverbeet (Swiss chard), spinach, spring onion (green part only), squash, swedes, sweet potato, taro, tomatoes, turnips, yams
MILK PRODUCTS _✗_	lactose-free milk, rice milk; 'hard' cheeses, including brie and camembert; lactose-free yoghurt; gelato and sorbets; butter and margarine _almond milk_
GRAIN FOODS _?_	gluten-free bread and cereal products, amaranth, arrowroot, buckwheat, corn (maize), millet, oats, polenta, potato, quinoa, rice, sorghum
SWEETENERS	sugar (sucrose), glucose, stevia, any other artificial sweeteners not ending in -ol (e.g. aspartame)
OTHER	garlic-infused oil as an onion and garlic substitute; fresh and dried herbs and spices, chives, ginger; maple syrup and golden syrup as honey substitutes

proteins - hummus (chickpeas & lentils & tofu & nut butters) (Fish & Seafood?)

→ Carbs, veg & protein.

Soluble fibre - no trigger.

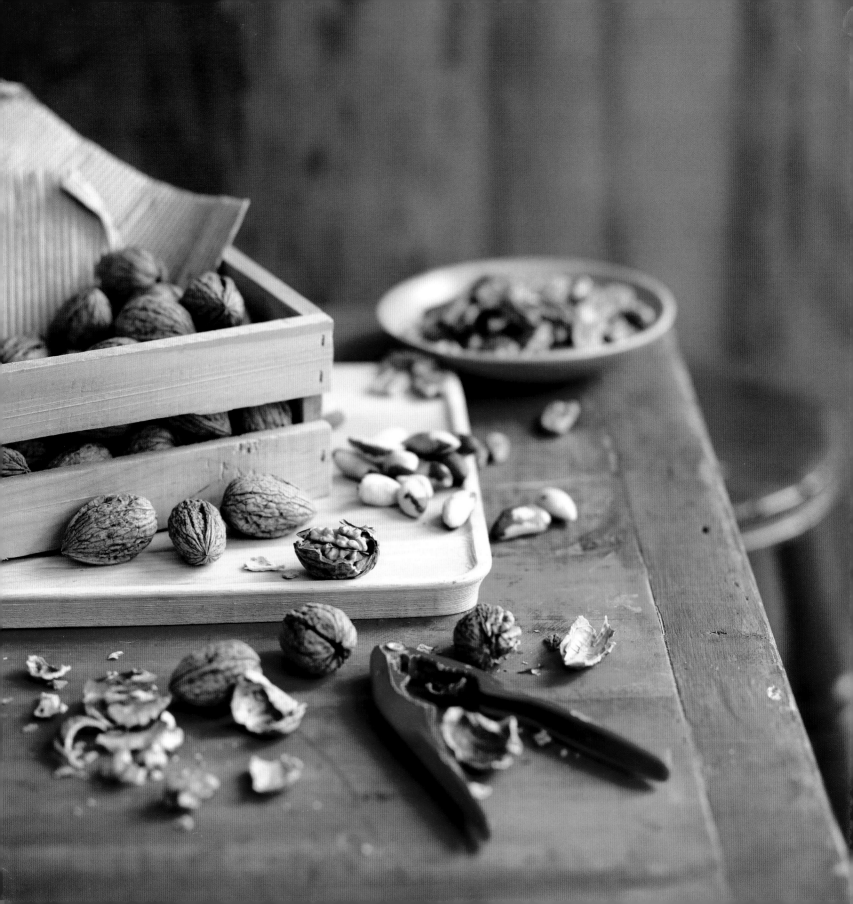

chapter four

Implementing the Low-FODMAP Diet

IF YOU'VE BEEN DIAGNOSED with IBS, or you've experienced bloating and abdominal discomfort with or without a change in your bowel habits, or you or your doctor believes you should follow the Low-FODMAP Diet, your first step should be to contact an Accredited Practising Dietitian who specialises in gastrointestinal nutrition.

That is not to say that the Low-FODMAP Diet is difficult to manage, but it will mean significant diet and lifestyle changes. You will have to learn about your condition, which foods are suitable and what will happen if you cease following the diet.

Where do I start?

To keep your symptoms under control, we recommend that you follow the Low-FODMAP Diet strictly by avoiding *all* FODMAPs, for at least two months. If your symptoms have improved after this time, you can, if desired, gradually reintroduce one FODMAP group at a time to see if you tolerate it. This is easier to do with the help of a specialist dietitian, who will review your symptoms and suggest the best approach, but for more on how to do it yourself, and fourteen days of menu plans, see pages 62–65.

Before you start the Low-FODMAP Diet, you may want to have a breath hydrogen test (see the box opposite), to see whether you have fructose or lactose malabsorption or both. If you discover that you don't have either, you will be able to include lactose and fructose in your Low-FODMAP Diet (i.e. a negative breath test for fructose and lactose does not mean you won't benefit from restricting the other remaining FODMAPs). If you decide not to have a breath test, we recommend you avoid *all* FODMAPs for the initial two months.

You may find many aspects of the Low-FODMAP Diet overwhelming at first. You will have to ask yourself these questions each morning: Where am I going to be today? Do I need to take food with me? Should I eat before I go? Will there be something there that I can eat? If you require a special diet, it can start to dictate your thoughts, and some people cope with this better than others. If you are having trouble adjusting, seek counselling or other assistance if you think it will help.

Here are some other important points to bear in mind when tailoring the Low-FODMAP Diet to your needs:

- *Consider all the FODMAP groups* – they all have the potential to cause bowel distension and other IBS symptoms.

- *No one can absorb fructans, GOS or polyols well* – which means you should always avoid them when first implementing the Low-FODMAP Diet.

- *Only some people have lactose or fructose malabsorption* – a breath hydrogen test will tell you whether or not you need to limit lactose or excess fructose in your diet.

- *Some FODMAPs cause more trouble in some people than others* – this depends on the proportions of each FODMAP in their diet, how well or poorly they absorb fructose and lactose, and how sensitive they are to each FODMAP, which could be related to which bacteria they have in their bowel. You'll get to know to which FODMAPs you are most sensitive.

BREATH HYDROGEN TESTS

Breath hydrogen tests are very useful to help plan a Low-FODMAP Diet.

Hydrogen is a gas that is produced by bacteria in the bowel when they ferment carbohydrates. Some of the hydrogen produced is absorbed across the lining of the large bowel into the bloodstream. The bloodstream then transports it to the lungs, where it is breathed out. Bacterial fermentation in the bowel is the *only* source of hydrogen gas in the breath. The same applies to the gas methane – in about 10 per cent of the population, the bacteria in the large bowel make methane rather than hydrogen. In a breath hydrogen test, we use a special instrument to measure the amount of hydrogen and methane gases breathed out from the lungs.

If you do the test, you will be asked to minimise your intake of fibre and FODMAPs in food for twenty-four hours beforehand so that there will be little if any hydrogen in the breath. You will also have to fast for several hours before the test. You will be asked to breathe into a bag or a handheld machine so that your breath sample can be taken. You will then be asked to drink a solution of a test sugar dissolved in water and breath samples will be taken every fifteen to twenty minutes for up to four hours.

Three sugars – lactulose, fructose and lactose – are usually tested. Lactulose cannot be digested or absorbed and is used to determine how vigorously your bacteria produce hydrogen and how fast the sugar travels out of the stomach and down the small intestine. Fructose and lactose are then tested. If your gut symptoms are triggered during or after the test, they will be noted down by the technician.

Any rise in the amount of hydrogen (or methane) in your breath after the sugar drink will mean that the sugar is being fermented by bacteria in your bowel and, therefore, that it is not completely absorbed. If fructose or lactose is completely absorbed (i.e. there is no rise in breath hydrogen), there is little need to restrict them in your diet. If your breath hydrogen does rise after you ingest fructose or lactose, then you should restrict them as part of your Low-FODMAP Diet.

although EFI recomends no. dairy

For more information on breath hydrogen tests and their interpretation, see this book's website, foodintolerancemanagementplan.com.au.

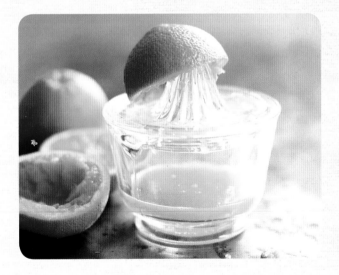

A Low-FODMAP Diet Q&A

Which FODMAPs should I avoid?

When you start the Low-FODMAP Diet you should avoid *all* FODMAPs – fructans, GOS, lactose, excess fructose and polyols. If you know you can completely absorb fructose, however, you need not restrict your excess fructose intake, and if you know you can completely absorb lactose, you need not restrict your lactose intake.

How much fruit can I eat at a time and how do I limit my fructose load?

You should eat no more than one serve of 'suitable' fruits (see page 35) per meal or sitting. One serve is usually one metric cup of cut-up fruit, or one whole piece of fruit, such as one orange or banana. You can enjoy many fruit serves each day, but you should allow two to three hours between each serve.

Can I eat 'table sugar'?

Table sugar (also called sucrose or cane sugar) should not cause symptoms if eaten in moderation. Sucrose is a double sugar made up of one part glucose and one part fructose. Large amounts of sucrose in one sitting may cause a problem for some people.

How do I balance my glucose and fructose intake?

If you need to avoid excess fructose, then consuming glucose at the same time as fructose could reduce the severity of your symptoms. You should be aware, however, that this strategy is not recommended if you have diabetes. Glucose sources include glucose powders and tablets, which are available in the sports-drink section of the supermarket and some health-food stores. How much glucose you need to consume with an excess of fructose will depend on how much of the food you are eating and what other foods you have recently consumed or are consuming at the same time. The best way is to use trial and error to establish how much glucose you require to remain free of IBS symptoms while consuming a food that has an excess of fructose.

Do I need to worry about fats and protein foods?

Fats and oils do not contain FODMAPs and nor do animal-based protein foods, such as meat, fish, chicken and eggs. However, plant-based protein foods such as legumes and lentils do contain FODMAPs and you may need to restrict your intake of these foods. FODMAPs typically occur in carbohydrate-based foods.

How do I avoid FODMAPs if I'm a vegetarian?

Vegetarians often consume large amounts of legumes as an important source of protein. However, these contain GOS and fructans. As there is a risk that your vegetarian or vegan diet will become nutritionally inadequate if you cut out legumes, your dietitian may advise you to allow a certain amount of these in your diet but exclude all other food sources of FODMAPs. The best approach will depend on your individual tolerance. For more tips on a vegetarian Low-FODMAP Diet, see page 52.

Must I really avoid wheat and rye products?

If you need to follow the Low-FODMAP Diet, you must avoid eating wheat and rye in large quantities. This means avoiding breads, cereals, pasta and biscuits, but you can still enjoy such things as a breadcrumb coating on a chicken schnitzel, or cookie pieces in ice cream. A specialist dietitian can help assess your individual intolerance to wheat and rye products. The table on the facing page gives common wheat-based products and suitable alternatives.

SUGGESTED ALTERNATIVES TO WHEAT-BASED FOODS

FOOD TYPE	WHEAT-BASED VARIETIES	SUGGESTED ALTERNATIVE
bread	white, wholemeal, multigrain and sourdough breads, mountain bread, pita bread, many 'rye breads'	gluten-free bread, oat bread, corn/maize tortillas or gluten-free flatbread _Spelt_
pasta and noodles	regular pasta, spelt pasta, most instant noodles, egg noodles (hokkien, udon), gnocchi	gluten-free pasta, rice noodles (vermicelli), wheat-free buckwheat (soba) noodles, — _LF_ mungbean (glass) noodles
breakfast cereals	most are made from wheat and may also contain excess dried fruit or have been sweetened with fruit juice	oat porridge, wheat-free muesli (with low fruit content), cornflakes, rice puffs, rice flakes, quinoa flakes, many gluten-free breakfast cereals _LF_
savoury biscuits	wheat-based varieties, water crackers	corn thins, rice cakes or crackers (but check for onion powder), gluten-free crackers, buckwheat crisp bread
cakes and baked goods	most are made from wheat	gluten-free cakes, flourless cakes, gluten-free baking mixes
sweet biscuits	wheat-based varieties	gluten-free biscuits, almond macaroons
pastry and breadcrumbs	made with wheat flour	gluten-free pastry mixes, gluten-free breadcrumbs (although wheat-based crumbs can usually be tolerated in small amounts), polenta, cornflake crumbs _LF_
other cereal products	semolina, couscous, bulgur	amaranth, buckwheat, chestnut, chia, corn (maize), millet, polenta, potato, quinoa, rice, sago, sorghum, tapioca and their flours

Rye products contain fructans and so should be restricted. Some people, however, find they can tolerate 100 per cent rye bread, probably because we can eat only small portions of it at a time. Some people may tolerate small amounts of 100 per cent spelt bread. Once you have been on the Low-FODMAP Diet for several weeks and your symptoms have improved, it might be worth trying small amounts of rye products to assess your own tolerance to them.

One bonus of a reduced-wheat diet is that you consume a greater variety of other grains, which means you can obtain a greater range of nutrients. An enormous variety of specialty gluten-free foods is now available, including delicious pasta, baking mixes, breakfast cereals, breads, biscuits and snack bars. You will find specialty gluten-free alternatives in the health-food aisle of your supermarket and in health-food stores. It's important to feel confident reading and interpreting food ingredient labels, and further guidance on this is provided on page 78.

Do I really need to avoid onions and garlic?

Onion is one of the greatest contributors to IBS symptoms. We recommend that you strictly avoid onion for at least two months. This means not only cooking without onion but also avoiding packaged foods that contain onion ingredients, such as onion powder in soups and stocks. You may find that you can reintroduce onion into your diet, but this will probably be only in very small amounts. If you cook with onion but leave it on your plate, this will only *reduce* the fructan load rather than remove it, since fructans can leach out of the onion into the other ingredients during cooking. Garlic also contains fructans, though if you like the flavour, one to two cloves per recipe can often be tolerated by IBS sufferers. An even better way to enjoy the taste of garlic without the fructans is to use garlic-infused oil – see page 78 for how to make it.

How do I know which foods I can eat?

The table below summarises foods that contain FODMAPs and suitable alternatives.

FODMAP-CONTAINING FOODS AND SUITABLE ALTERNATIVES

FOOD TYPE	VARIETIES CONTAINING FODMAPS	SUITABLE ALTERNATIVES
flours and grains	wheat and legume products, including bulgur, chickpea flour (besan),* couscous, durum, kumat, lentil flour,* multigrain flour, pea flour,* rye, semolina, soy flour,* triticale, wheat bran, wheat flour, wheaten cornflour, wheatgerm	arrowroot, barley, buckwheat flour, cornflour and cornmeal (maize), custard powder, glutinous rice, ground rice, malt, oat bran, oatmeal, oats, polenta, potato flour, quinoa, rice (brown, white), rice bran, rice flour, sago, tapioca, wild rice
cereals	wheat-based and mixed-grain breakfast cereals, bulgur, couscous, muesli, semolina	rice- or corn-based breakfast cereals, rolled oats (porridge), baby rice cereal, wheat-free muesli (with minimal amounts of suitable dried fruit) ▶

* These contain GOS and fructans, but in small amounts as part of a recipe, do not cause IBS symptoms in most people. You should assess your own tolerance.

FOOD TYPE	VARIETIES CONTAINING FODMAPS	SUITABLE ALTERNATIVES
pasta and noodles	noodles, pasta, spatlese, gnocchi	mungbean (glass) noodles, rice noodles, rice vermicelli, soba noodles, gluten-free pasta
breads, biscuits and cakes	all breads, biscuits, cakes, muffins, croissants, crumpets and pastries containing wheat and rye; sourdough commercial breads; breadcrumbs	gluten-free breads, taco shells, maize tortillas, plain rice cakes and crackers, gluten-free biscuits, gluten-free cakes and pastries
dairy foods and alternatives	regular milk, ice cream, soft cheeses (in large quantities), yoghurt	lactose-free milk, calcium-fortified soy milk,* lactose-free ice cream, hard cheeses, most lactose-free yoghurts, tofu*
meat and equivalents	sausages and other smallgoods (check for onion and dehydrated vegetable powders)	plain red meat, fish, poultry, bacon, eggs
nuts and seeds		all nuts and seeds
fruit and vegetables	see lists on pages 26, 32–33	see list on page 35
spreads and condiments	most commercial relishes, chutneys, onion-containing gravies, stock cubes, dressings and sauces, honey	jam, marmalade, golden syrup, maple syrup, peanut butter, soy sauce, tamari, vinegar (see page 35)
beverages	coffee substitutes; large quantities of fruit juice; apple, pear and mango juices	water, rice milk, mineral water, soda water, soft drinks, tonic water, fruit juice (safe fruits only, 125 ml per serve), tea, coffee, most alcohols (see list on pages 49–50)
fats and oils	large amounts of margarine and dairy whip/table spread	vegetable oils, butter, ghee, lard, dripping, small serves of cream
others		baking powder, bicarbonate of soda, cocoa, gelatine, pure icing sugar, salt, xanthan gum, herbs, spices (see page 35)

* Soy milk and tofu are usually well tolerated. Assess your individual tolerance.

Are there other ways to tackle lactose malabsorption?
If you have lactose malabsorption, you can buy lactase enzyme in tablets or drops in pharmacies and some health-food stores. The enzyme will break down the lactose in lactose-containing food and beverages so that you can absorb it. This may help enhance variety in your diet and make it easier for you when eating away from home. Take lactase tablets at the same time as the lactose-containing food or drink – refer to the packet for how many to take. Add lactase drops to a lactose-containing fluid twenty-four hours before you intend to drink it.

Reintroducing the FODMAPs one at a time

All FODMAPs can cause IBS symptoms, and if they are eaten together, their effect is cumulative. Any meal is likely to contain a variety of foods and, therefore, a complex mixture of carbohydrates, which includes FODMAPs. The Low-FODMAP Diet aims to reduce the intake of *all* FODMAPs so that IBS symptoms are reduced as much as possible.

While all FODMAPs are potential triggers for IBS symptoms, which FODMAP has the greatest effect on you will depend on how much and how often you consume foods that contain them. In Australia, fructose and fructans are by far the most widespread and frequently eaten FODMAPs. Lactose, GOS and polyol intake can vary significantly across the population. Intake can also vary seasonally – sorbitol intake is likely to be higher in summer when stone fruits are in abundance. Indian and Mexican cuisines, which are based largely on lentils and beans, will have a higher GOS content.

Once you have followed the Low-FODMAP Diet for two months and seen an improvement in your symptoms, you can consider re-introducing the FODMAPs one at a time, to determine which contribute to your symptoms and how much of each you can tolerate. This process is called a food challenge. Here are some guidelines for FODMAP food challenges.

1. Test only one FODMAP subgroup at a time. (Use the suggestions in the flowchart to the right.)

2. Choose an amount of FODMAP that reflects a normal intake. You will gain no useful information about your tolerance of a FODMAP group if you challenge yourself with a very large intake in your trial dose. Any food consumed in excessive amounts is likely to induce symptoms.

3. Where possible, choose a food that contains only one type of FODMAP, to enable a more accurate interpretation of your response.

4. Continue to restrict *all* other FODMAPs until your tolerance (or intolerance) is confirmed.

5. Maintain a consistent intake of caffeine and alcohol, or of any other foods you know are a problem for you.

6. Challenge with one FODMAP per week.

7. Eat the challenge food at least twice during the test week (or until symptoms are triggered).

Monitor your symptom response.
   If you don't get symptoms
   - increase the number of foods that contain the FODMAP you are testing, and assess your response; *or*
   - maintain the amount and type of food you have tested, and then undertake the next FODMAP challenge.
   If you do get symptoms
   - wait until you are symptom free, then reduce the serving size to half and challenge again; *or*

- assume the FODMAP is a problem for you. It is recommended to continue to restrict the FODMAP and follow the suggestions below.
  - Try another food from within the same FODMAP group to confirm the result of the challenge.
  - The **dose** of FODMAPs is vital when challenging foods. We suggest you halve the amount of food and try again when you are symptom free. It is unlikely you will have to omit the FODMAP completely.
  - We encourage you to challenge again in the future as your sensitivity to FODMAPs may change over time.

A suggested order, type and quantity of food for the reintroduction of each FODMAP subgroup are shown in the flowchart. The order is a guide only – choose an order that works for you.

FODMAP REINTRODUCTION PLAN

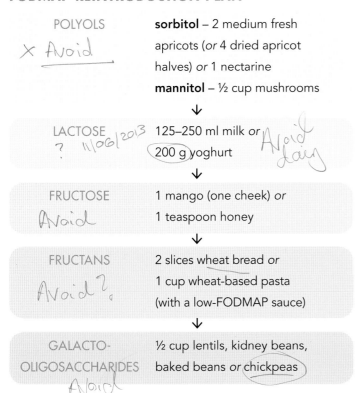

POLYOLS	**sorbitol** – 2 medium fresh apricots (*or* 4 dried apricot halves) *or* 1 nectarine **mannitol** – ½ cup mushrooms
LACTOSE	125–250 ml milk *or* 200 g yoghurt
FRUCTOSE	1 mango (one cheek) *or* 1 teaspoon honey
FRUCTANS	2 slices wheat bread *or* 1 cup wheat-based pasta (with a low-FODMAP sauce)
GALACTO-OLIGOSACCHARIDES	½ cup lentils, kidney beans, baked beans *or* chickpeas

What if the Low-FODMAP Diet doesn't work for me?

Although the Low-FODMAP Diet is very effective, it is not a panacea – for about one in four people it has little, if any, effect on IBS symptoms, although this is often because they are not being absolutely strict about following the diet. You must be dedicated to the diet; being selective about what you restrict won't work. For a small proportion of IBS sufferers, diet itself is not a factor. Some, for instance, swallow too much air or their gut handles poorly any air they swallow. Such people need to avoid fizzy drinks and gulping of liquids, and perhaps need to work on anxiety issues using psychological support – from relaxation techniques and yoga to cognitive behaviour therapy and hypnotherapy. There is evidence that hypnotherapy can help reduce the symptoms of IBS in the long term. The Australian Hypnotherapy Association has a list of members who are IBS-trained.

It may be that other food components are the triggers for your IBS symptoms. Some people have tried wider carbohydrate restriction through elimination of resistant starch and fibre as well as the FODMAPs, and reducing the intake of foods containing bioactive chemicals, such as salicylates, amines and glutamates. If you are considering taking this approach, we recommend you do so only under the supervision of a specialist dietitian, otherwise you may not be getting all the nutrients you need.

Another approach is to abandon the FODMAP restriction and undertake an elimination diet, followed by a food-rechallenge process. This method is time-consuming and tedious. It should be attempted only under the supervision of an allergy specialist and/or specialist dietitian. While skin, blood and other tests may help identify food hypersensitivities, their interpretation requires the expertise of an allergy specialist.

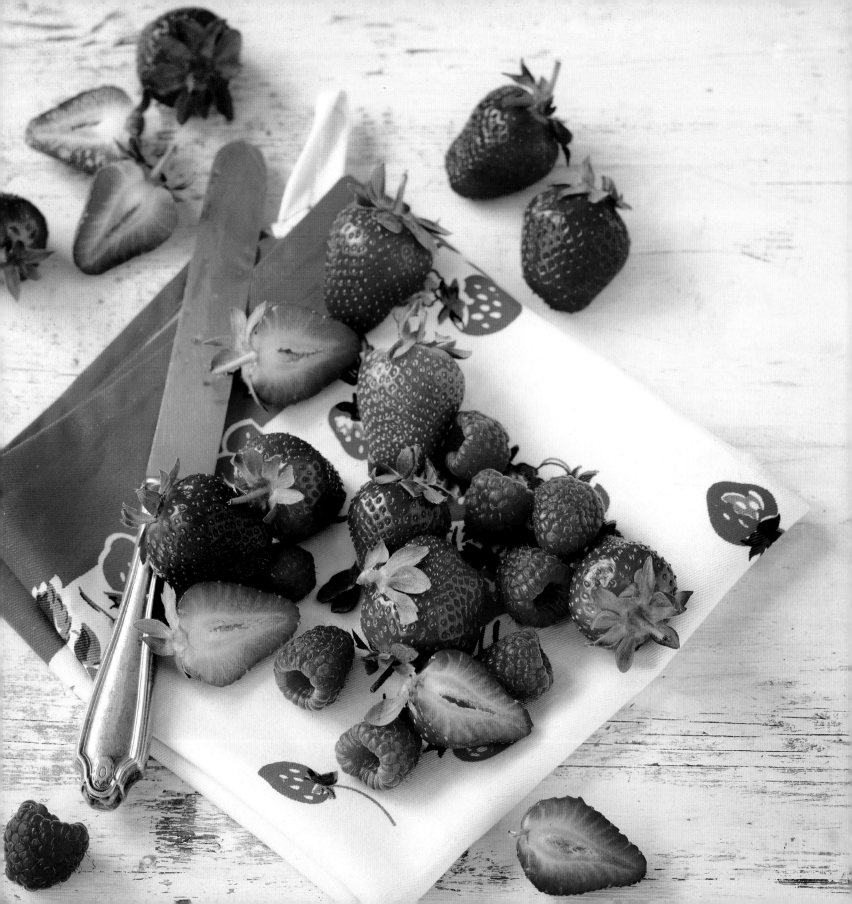

chapter five

Putting the Low-FODMAP Diet into practice

THIS CHAPTER will help you manage the Low-FODMAP Diet, whether for an average day at work or home, or a social occasion. There is information on snacks, drinks, how to adapt the recipes in your cookbooks (although there are plenty of delicious recipes in this book!), baking hints and tips for vegetarians, diabetics, people with inflammatory bowel disease, and children. For easy menu plans, go to the next chapter. And for tips on equipping your kitchen, low-FODMAP shopping and flavouring your food, go to Chapter 7.

Snacks

It would be a waste of hard work if you followed the Low-FODMAP Diet conscientiously at mealtimes but then ate unsuitable high-FODMAP snacks in between. Here are some great low-FODMAP snack ideas:

- *Fruit* – fresh fruit makes an excellent snack. See the table on page 35 for suitable fruits and limit yourself to one piece or small handful at a time.

- *Vegetables* – vegetable pieces such as raw carrot, celery, capsicum (pepper), cucumber sticks, tomatoes, cherry tomatoes or corn on the cob.

- *Dry biscuits* – gluten-free crisp bread, rice cakes, rice crackers (no onion powder) or corn thins with one of the toppings or cheeses below.

- *Toppings* – peanut butter, red meat, chicken, fish, egg, cheese, grated or sliced vegetables, creamed corn and a small serve of cottage cheese.

- *Cheese* – hard cheeses (see page 31), cheese sticks, cheese triangles, cheese slices or mini cheeses.

- *Other 'every day' treats* – yoghurt (lactose-free if necessary), popcorn, mixed nuts, nut and seed mixes (e.g. pepitas and sunflower seeds) or a boiled egg.

- *Homemade 'sometimes' treats* – try the following recipes from this book:

  - *Cakes* – Basic Chocolate Cake (page 191), Vanilla Cake (page 194), Carrot and Pecan Cake (page 197), Sweet Chestnut Cake (page 208), Moist Banana Cake (page 207).

  - *Muffins* – Pineapple Muffins (page 205), Chia Seed and Spice Muffins (page 203).

  - *Biscuits* – Simple Sweet Biscuits (page 190), Choc Chip Biscuits (page 186), Macaroons (page 186).

  - *Slices* – Lemon Lime Slice (page 199), Strawberry Slice (page 230).

  - *Baked savoury treats* – Chilli Capsicum Cornbread (page 181), Zucchini and Pepita Cornmeal Bread (page 182).

  - *Other baked sweet treats* – Sultana Scones (page 188), Lemon Friands (page 201).

- *Commercial 'sometimes' treats* – chocolate, potato crisps (no onion powder), lollies, ice cream (lactose-free if necessary).

The 'sometimes' foods should remain a small contribution to the diet against the background of a nutritious eating plan.

Non-alcoholic beverages

- *Water* – is the best drink! Drink water in preference to all other drinks, and without restriction. You may like to squeeze lemon or lime juice into the water for a flavour twist.

- *Cordial* – the fruit content of cordials, even 60 per cent or more fruit-juice cordials, is not a problem for the Low-FODMAP Diet.

- *Soft drinks* – these are typically sweetened with sucrose in Australia and are suitable for a Low-FODMAP Diet. In some countries (especially the USA), however, they are sweetened with high-fructose corn syrup, and should be avoided. Bear in mind that if you consume large quantities of sucrose-sweetened soft drinks, you may also be consuming a high fructose load. Ideally, you should restrict sucrose-sweetened soft drinks to 250 ml per sitting to limit your fructose load. Diet soft drinks are suitable for the Low-FODMAP Diet.

- *Dairy-alternative drinks* – including rice milk, oat milk, almond milk and quinoa milk. These can be consumed freely as they are lactose-free and low-FODMAP. Soy milks are usually well tolerated.

- *Sports drinks* – the sweeteners used in electrolyte drinks vary. If they are sweetened with fructose, they should be avoided. Check the ingredients to determine if they are suitable for you to consume, and be mindful about how much you drink at once.

- *Fruit juices* – if these are made from suitable fruits (e.g. orange, cranberry, pineapple or tomato), they are suitable for the Low-FODMAP Diet, but should still be consumed only in small amounts, typically 125 ml in one sitting. Any more than this may contribute to an excess fructose load. Many fruit-based drinks may include apple or pear juice, even if this isn't indicated in the name of the product. Always read the ingredients of fruit-based beverages to ensure there are no surprise high-FODMAP ingredients.

- *Vegetable juices* – if these are freshly prepared using suitable vegetables, you can drink freely on the Low-FODMAP Diet. Many commercially prepared vegetable juices, however, contain onion and should be avoided. Many also use tomato juice. If a vegetable juice is tomato-based, limit the quantity to 125 ml.

- *Dandelion tea* – this contains fructans and should therefore be avoided or consumed only in limited quantities according to your own degree of tolerance.

- *Chicory-based (coffee-substitute) drinks* – these are typically made using inulin from the dried root of chicory plants and are high-FODMAP drinks. You should avoid them, or consume them only in limited quantities according to your own degree of tolerance.

Alcoholic beverages

GENERAL RECOMMENDATIONS

Alcoholic beverages should always be enjoyed only in moderation, but if you have IBS this is even more important, as alcohol in excess can aggravate an irritable bowel. You don't need to avoid alcohol completely, but a sensible, moderate approach will enable you to enjoy a social drink without inducing your IBS symptoms. If you consume alcoholic beverages with food, they are less likely to induce IBS symptoms than if you drink on an empty stomach. This is because the food slows down the release of alcohol from the stomach.

Alcoholic drinks can stimulate your appetite and tend to make you more relaxed. Under these conditions, you may be less likely to adhere to the Low-FODMAP Diet as strictly as you should. If you wish to consume alcohol, the recommendations are one standard drink for women, and two standard drinks for men per day, with two alcohol-free days per week.

ALCOHOLIC BEVERAGES AND THE LOW-FODMAP DIET

A potential problem with alcohol is its fructose load.

- *Wine* – this varies in its sweetness. A dry wine contains minimal sugar and is not a problem, but sweet wines are probably best avoided – check the label for clues. Watch out particularly for dessert wines, often referred to as 'stickies', especially since they are often consumed with sweet food, which further contributes to the fructose load. Examples include fortified wines such as port, marsala, madeira, vermouth, liqueurs, muscat and tokay, and unfortified dessert wines such as botrytis dessert wines, rice wine and sauterne.

- *Beer* – this presents a different problem. Beer contains the FODMAP mannitol. While the amount of mannitol in beer may not be high, beer is often drunk in large quantities in one sitting, which leads to a large dose of mannitol. Although some types of beer are made from wheat, only a small amount of the wheat remains and is not a problem. Beer, ale, lager, stout and Guinness, which all contain gluten, are not suitable for people with coeliac disease but are suitable for people on the Low-FODMAP Diet if consumed in very modest proportions.

- *Spirits* – these do not contain FODMAPs, even if they are originally derived from wheat or rye. Spirits on their own are suitable for a Low-FODMAP Diet, but do not consume large quantities because excessive alcohol intake can aggravate the symptoms of IBS. The bigger risk with spirits is usually the mixer.

- *Mixers* – these are usually sugar-sweetened drinks (soft drinks) or juices (such as orange, lime or cranberry juice). Most mixers have balanced fructose and glucose, but beware of some, such as US soft drinks, which may be sweetened with high-fructose corn syrup. Alternatively, you can use a 'diet' soft drink. Occasionally milk is used as the mixer, which may be a problem if you have lactose malabsorption. The problem with most mixers lies in the total fructose load if they are consumed in excess. A good rule is to limit your intake to two glasses per sitting.

- *Other alcoholic beverages* – the ones to watch out for are 'coolers' and cider. A cooler is a low-alcohol drink made from white or red wine mixed with a soft drink, soda or juice. Treat them as if they are a fruit juice or soft drink and limit your intake to two glasses per sitting. Cider, an alcoholic beverage typically based on apple juice, is unsuitable for the Low-FODMAP Diet.

Main meal substitutions

This book includes a range of great-tasting low-FODMAP recipes that you, your friends and the whole family can enjoy. You might also like to adapt one of your own favourite recipes so that it is low in FODMAPs. One easy example is changing a quiche recipe to a pastryless frittata. If you are not confident that packaged foods are low-FODMAP, cook your meals using basic unprocessed ingredients. Information about low-FOD-MAP recipe books and shopping guides is included on this book's website, foodintolerancemanagementplan.com.au.

We recommend that if you share meals with other members of your household, you serve everyone the same low-FODMAP dishes. The other members of your household will still be able to enjoy high-FODMAP foods for breakfast and lunch, but you will save time, confusion and dirty dishes if you don't cook two separate dinners. The Low-FODMAP Diet is not a bland, tasteless diet at all. If you miss onion, see the tips on page 78 for boosting the flavour of your food.

Basic baking tips

No single flour can be substituted directly for wheat flour. None has the same excellent texture, elasticity and nice feeling in the mouth. A combination of wheat-free flours (usually three or more) works best, since different flours contribute different properties. A good wheat-free flour blend is:

- 2 parts rice flour (fine)

- 1 part soy flour (debittered)*

- 1 part either potato flour or cornflour (maize cornstarch) or tapioca flour

Use the table overleaf to adapt your baking to your low-FODMAP needs. Baking without wheat flour presents more challenges for the chef, but the following tips should make baking more successful:

- Xanthan gum, guar gum and CMC (carboxymethyl cellulose) can be used as a 'gluten substitute' to help improve the elasticity and crumb structure of baked goods. They can also assist in moisture retention. They are readily available in health-food stores. As a general guide, add xanthan gum as follows: breads – 1 heaped teaspoon; cakes – 1 teaspoon; biscuits – ½ teaspoon; muffins – 1 teaspoon; pastry – 1 teaspoon.

- Use a variety of flours and sift them together three times to ensure even mixing and aeration. Sift any raising agents (such as baking powder and bicarbonate of soda) and vegetable gums together with the flours.

* These contain GOS and fructans, but in small amounts as part of a recipe, do not cause IBS symptoms in most people. Assess your own tolerance.

SOME SUGGESTED LOW-FODMAP FLOUR MIXES

FOOD TYPE	FINE RICE FLOUR	CORNFLOUR (MAIZE)	POTATO FLOUR	TAPIOCA FLOUR	SOY FLOUR*	COMMENT
cake 1	2 parts	1 part			1 part	may substitute potato or tapioca flour for the maize cornflour
cake 2	2 parts	1 part	1 part			increase the quantity of eggs for binding and for protein
biscuits	3 parts	2 parts			1 part	fine rice flour is important for texture
pastry	2 parts	1 part			1 part	add xanthan gum to improve elasticity and assist in rolling
scones		2 parts		2 parts	1 part	tapioca flour is important for texture

* These contain GOS and fructans, but in small amounts as part of a recipe, do not cause IBS symptoms in most people. You should assess your own tolerance.

- Wheat-free baked goods (with the exception of those made using almond or hazelnut meals) tend to dry out more quickly than wheat-based goods, so it's a good idea to cut cakes into slices and freeze the excess portions or to make muffins instead. They will defrost well, but if your gluten-free baked goods seem dry or stale, rejuvenate them in a microwave for 20–30 seconds on high.

- Use baking paper to line your cake tins and biscuit trays, and roll your wheat-free pastry between two sheets of baking paper.

- Wheat-free baking is often less forgiving, so make sure you follow the recipe to the letter. For the best results, ensure your oven temperature is accurate and follow the suggested cooking times.

The Low-FODMAP Diet for vegetarians

A carefully constructed vegetarian diet can be very healthy, but it does require some extra planning. Vegetarians, and particularly vegans, need to be careful about getting enough protein and other nutrients, so should include a wide range of nutritious foods and supplements to provide essential nutrients, some of which, like vitamin B12, occur only in animal foods.

LEGUMES AND OLIGOSACCHARIDES

In a vegetarian diet, GOS and fructans are often consumed in large quantities as a key source of protein, particularly for vegans. These may include: chickpeas, dry beans (kidney, haricot, pinto, navy, lima, butter, adzuki, mung and broad beans), lentils, lupins and soybeans.

SOY PRODUCTS AND THE LOW-FODMAP DIET

The soy-related FODMAPs that occur in tofu, tempeh, miso and soy milk, soy yoghurt and soy cheese are generally tolerated well by people following the Low-FODMAP Diet, but this is not always predictable. We suggest that you include soy products in your diet for their nutritional importance, and then monitor your tolerance to them. In other words, you need to determine your own threshold of tolerance. If you *can* tolerate these, then you can include soy and other legumes. If you are an ovo-lacto vegetarian and intolerant to legumes and soy-based foods, you will be able to avoid them without compromising your protein intake by consuming adequate amounts of milk- and egg-based foods. If you are vegan and intolerant to legumes and soy-based foods, you may find it difficult to meet your daily protein needs. Nuts and seeds, cereal products based on high-protein grains and cereals, and protein-enriched milk alternatives will be your most significant protein sources. Make a conscious effort to eat them in sufficient quantities.

TIPS FOR ENSURING AN ADEQUATE PROTEIN INTAKE

- Eat nuts and seeds daily, nibbling them as a snack or enjoying nut or seed spreads such as peanut butter and tahini.

- Choose low-FODMAP protein-enriched milk substitutes such as protein-enriched rice, oat, almond and quinoa milks.

- Choose cereal-based foods such as pasta, breakfast cereals, breads and crispbreads made from high-protein ingredients such as quinoa, amaranth and chia.

- If legumes are not tolerated, include the 'better tolerated' soy products such as soy milk, textured vegetable protein and tofu.

- If you eat dairy, include milk and yoghurt (lactose-free if necessary), and cheese.

- If you eat eggs, eat at least two serves per week.

- Every day, eat wholegrain cereal foods such as grainy low-FODMAP bread or breakfast cereal, quinoa, amaranth and chia.

We recommend that you consult an Accredited Practising Dietitian if you are vegan and wish to follow the Low-FODMAP Diet. Without professional advice, it will be difficult to ensure an adequate intake of vitamin B12 and protein, and to maintain your energy levels. There are sample vegetarian and vegan Low-FODMAP Diet menu plans in the next chapter.

The Low-FODMAP Diet and diabetes

Both IBS and diabetes rely on a specialised diet for good health, and the Low-FODMAP Diet is ideal for both. Below are some Low-FODMAP tips for those with diabetes.

- Eat regular meals and snacks and keep the size of your meals moderate. Try not to overeat.

- Eat a variety of foods at each mealtime. Include a carbohydrate source, such as wheat-free bread and cereals, pasta, corn, sweet potato or rice; a protein source, such as lean red meat, fish, chicken or eggs; and plenty of appropriate vegetables at each meal.

- Limit high-fat foods, especially those containing saturated fat, such as the skin on chicken, fat on meat, butter, full-fat dairy foods, cheese, cream, coconut milk, takeaway foods and processed meats.

- Avoid trying to balance fructose with glucose to assist with fructose absorption.

- Limit your alcohol intake. Two standard drinks for men and one standard drink for women per day are the recommended maximums for good health. Have at least two alcohol-free days a week.

DIABETES AND THE GLYCAEMIC INDEX

A diet for the management of diabetes attempts to control blood glucose levels and maintain a healthy weight. The regularity of meals and the amount eaten are important, as is the choice of foods. To assist with that choice, a ranking system of foods called the glycaemic index (GI) has been devised.

The GI ranks foods containing carbohydrate according to how much they raise blood glucose levels. In order to test a food's GI, we monitor a test subject's blood glucose levels every fifteen minutes during a two-hour period after they have eaten a known amount of the food. The higher a food's GI, the faster the blood glucose levels rise, and their peak level will be higher than that caused by a low-GI food. The lower a food's GI, the slower the blood glucose levels rise when it is eaten. This represents a slower but more sustained blood glucose response, which is important for diabetes control.

Although we rarely eat one food at a time, the lower the GI of each of the food components making up the meal, the lower the meal's total GI will tend to be. Many factors affect GI, including dietary fibre content, the degree to which the grains have been processed, the molecular structure of the starch and the presence of fat.

THE GI OF LOW-FODMAP FOODS

Many low-GI foods have too many FODMAPs in them and are therefore not suitable for the Low-FODMAP Diet. This applies particularly to wheat-based wholegrain foods such as wholegrain breads and pasta. Although wheat-free substitutes can have a higher GI, dairy products and many fresh fruits and vegetables have a low GI. Most of these are suitable for the Low-FODMAP Diet.

LOW-GI TIPS

- Include one low-GI food with each meal to lower the overall GI of the meal, such as (lactose-free) yoghurt, suitable low-FODMAP fruit, amaranth, chia, quinoa, LSA mix or rice bran with your breakfast cereal.

- Choose foods that are less processed with lots of low-FODMAP whole grains and fibre.

- Add seeds, nuts and chia to homemade breads.

- Cook your wheat-free pasta al dente (firm to the bite) – this will lower the GI.

- Eat in moderation – even if a food has a low GI, eating too much of it will have a significant effect on your blood glucose.

- Try to limit juices and soft drinks – not only are they not suitable in large amounts for the Low-FODMAP Diet, they can also contribute to high blood sugar levels.

- Some low-GI foods may be high in fat or kilojoules and are therefore not a suitable regular addition to your diet.

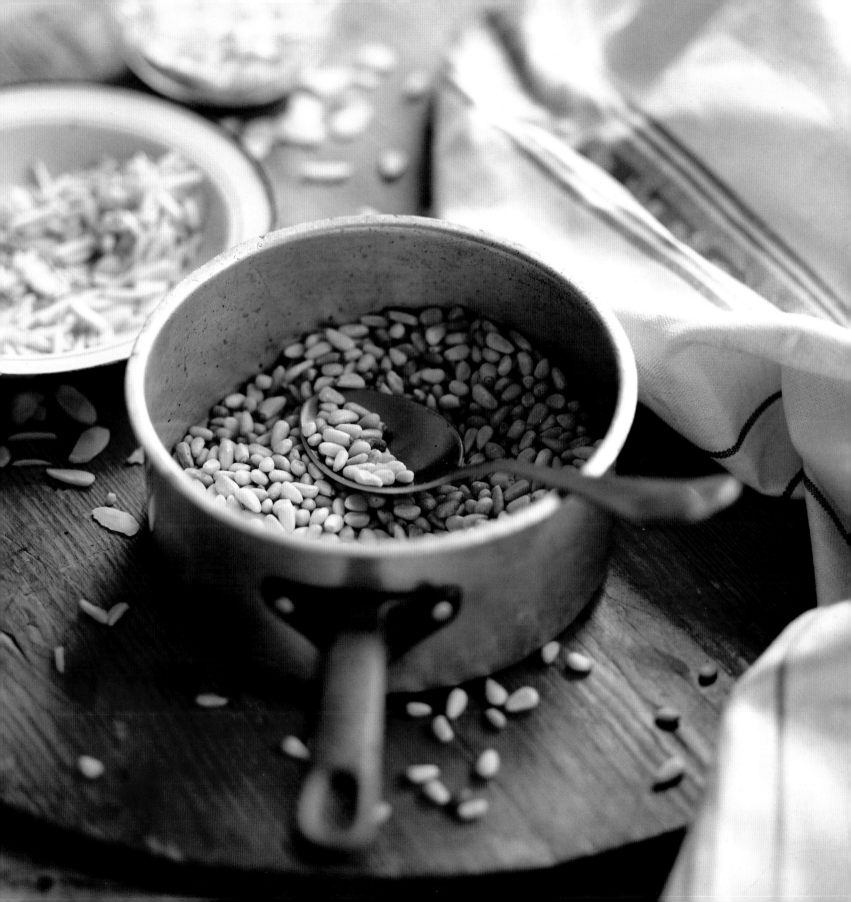

The Low-FODMAP Diet and coeliac disease

The gluten-free diet is the only treatment for people with coeliac disease, and it must be strictly followed for life. This should not only help improve the condition of the small bowel lining, but also other aspects of health, including gastrointestinal symptoms. Some people may follow the gluten-free diet strictly but still experience ongoing gastrointestinal symptoms; in this case, then IBS may be occurring at the same time as coeliac disease.

If this is the case with you, we recommend that you first consult an Accredited Practising Dietitian, to confirm that you are not accidentally ingesting any gluten. It can be difficult to know all sources of gluten that may be present in foods. A dietitian is trained to know all the hidden sources, and may identify some that could be the cause of your symptoms. If, however, they conclude that you have been following a strict gluten-free diet, then you are likely to benefit from trying the Low-FODMAP Diet in combination with the gluten-free diet to reduce your gastrointestinal symptoms.

People with coeliac disease may choose to allow some FODMAP-containing foods in their diet after their initial trial – this is acceptable, as FODMAPs will not cause damage to the body if consumed. The gluten free-diet, however, must remain strict at all times.

Although gluten-free foods are (generally) wheat-free, not all gluten-free foods are Low FODMAP – for example, a gluten-free apple pie. Although absolute avoidance of wheat is not necessary for people following only the Low-FODMAP Diet (they can, for example, eat breadcrumbs), this is *not* the case for people with coeliac disease – wheat-derived ingredients containing detectable gluten (including regular breadcrumbs) must be strictly avoided at all times.

See the description of wheat ingredients on page 41. If you have coeliac disease and wish to follow the Low-FODMAP Diet, we strongly recommend that you consult an Accredited Practising Dietitian. Without professional advice, it may be difficult to ensure a nutritionally adequate intake. All of the recipes in this book are gluten-free.

The Low-FODMAP Diet and inflammatory bowel disease

Inflammatory bowel disease (often known as IBD) is an illness in which the bowel becomes chronically inflamed. This may cause diarrhoea (that can be bloody), abdominal pain, tiredness and many other symptoms. There are two main types of IBD, Crohn's disease (which can affect any part of the gut) and ulcerative colitis (which affects only the large bowel). The causes for these conditions are not known, and treatment is directed towards controlling the inflammation and preventing it from returning. Dietary change plays only a very small role in this aspect of treatment.

Many people with IBD may benefit in other ways from dietary change. For example, when the IBD is active, some people may require a temporary change to their usual dietary intake, such as a low-residue diet (if there is narrowing in the bowel) or a high-protein/energy diet (if there is poor absorption and/or weight loss).

Loose bowel motions, bloating, wind and pain frequently occur at times when the IBD is active, but these symptoms can also be common even when the bowel inflammation is well controlled. Our studies have shown that the Low-FODMAP Diet effectively reduces these symptoms when the inflammation has been successfully treated. Our research has also shown that fructose and lactose malabsorption are more common in people with IBD than in the general population.

If you have IBD but also experience symptoms of IBS, we suggest you implement the Low-FODMAP Diet. In our experience it offers relief to most sufferers.

The Low-FODMAP Diet for children

Raising children with food intolerances is most successful when the parents spend time explaining the situation to the child and their siblings, and get them actively involved in making food choices and finding suitable alternatives. Fortunately, it is much easier these days for children to follow a therapeutic diet, as there are so many different foods catering for a wide variety of special dietary needs.

Peer pressure can pose challenges, so it's important to educate your child's friends and teachers too. There is an increased awareness in schools these days of the needs of children with food allergies and intolerances. Special diets are generally well incorporated and the whole class is usually very accepting.

Children should never restrict foods from their diet unless they have a confirmed food intolerance or allergy.

TIPS FOR SCHOOL CAMPS

- Teachers and camp organisers usually have a protocol for managing special cases, including dietary requirements. If they are already aware of your child's needs, they may approach you before you need to approach them.

- Even if you have already explained your child's diet to their teacher, you may need to refresh their memory. Make sure no questions are left unanswered and that the teachers are confident about your child's needs.

- Talk to the camp cook and check the menu. Work out suitable alternatives (taking into account limitations such as food availability, cost and time).

- Provide cereal, bread, snacks and so on if necessary, or tell the organisers where to purchase them. Work out an arrangement regarding the cost of the camp if you provide a large quantity of food, bearing in mind that flexibility in pricing may not be possible in some situations.

- Encourage the camp organisers to contact you if they have *any* concerns about your child's diet. It is preferable for this to occur 'behind the scenes', so that your child's diet doesn't become the major focus of the camp either for your child or the other children.

- Train your child to choose appropriate foods and if in doubt to leave them out. They should be able to manage quite well.

- Do what you can to prevent your child from having FODMAP foods, but remember that accidents will happen. Your child should be allowed to enjoy the camp, and the socialisation of eating.

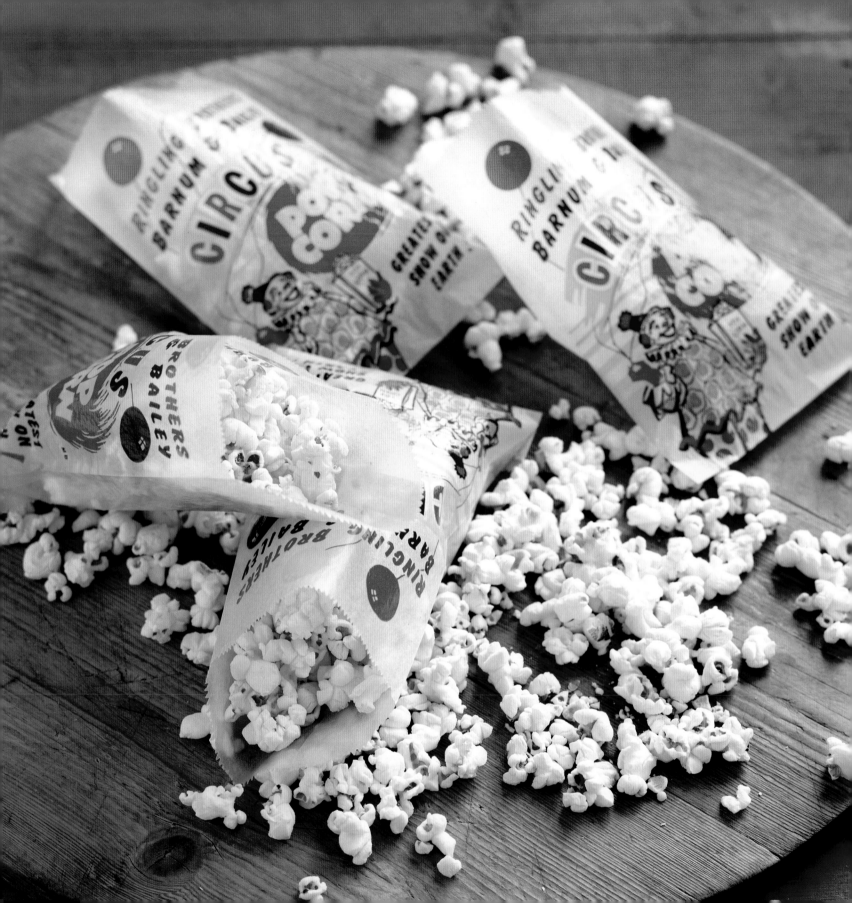

TIPS FOR PARTIES

- Where possible, ask the host parents what will be served at the party. If you have time, prepare low-FODMAP equivalents for the host parents to reheat and serve at the same time.

- If possible, suggest low-FODMAP ingredients for those dishes the host parents intend to prepare.

- Find out what flavour the birthday cake is and give your child a slice of a similarly flavoured cake to take so they can eat with the others. Bear in mind, however, that your child will probably tolerate a small 'wheat breakout'.

- Work with your child's needs. If your child is happy to have their own pack of favourite foods irrespective of what the other children are eating, then that may be a simpler solution for all concerned.

TIPS FOR SLEEPOVERS

- Explain your child's diet to the host family. See how much they wish to contribute, how adaptable they are and go from there.

- Pack extra snacks in your child's school lunch so that they will have something to munch on straight after school at the host's house.

- Give the host parents guidelines about suitable dinner options. A simple meal of 'meat and vegetables' is acceptable for most families, and will suit your child.

- Check out the type of cereal usually offered by the host family. If it is unsuitable, pack a serve of cereal for your child to take, and some lactose-free milk if lactose intolerant.

- As the host parents become more familiar with your child's needs, you may need to prepare less each time and you may be able to buy packets of your child's breakfast cereal and bread to keep on hand.

TIPS FOR LUNCHBOXES

- Cold roast red meats, chicken or eggs with salad.

- Wheat-free sandwiches, or bread alternatives such as rice cakes, rice crisp breads or corn thins, filled with cold meat and cheese or peanut butter (if permitted).

- Vegetable sticks and/or plain corn chips and dip.

- Yoghurt or fromage frais (lactose-free if necessary).

- A slice of wheat-free pizza.

- Quiche (made using wheat-free pastry or a rice crust), a slice of frittata (see page 113), polenta wedges (see page 127) or omelette wraps.

- Sushi and sashimi, fried rice (onion-free), rice balls (arancini) or rice-paper rolls.

- Fresh fruit (whole or cut into pieces).

- Boiled eggs.

- Plain popcorn or savoury muffins.

- Leftovers from last night's low-FODMAP dinner.

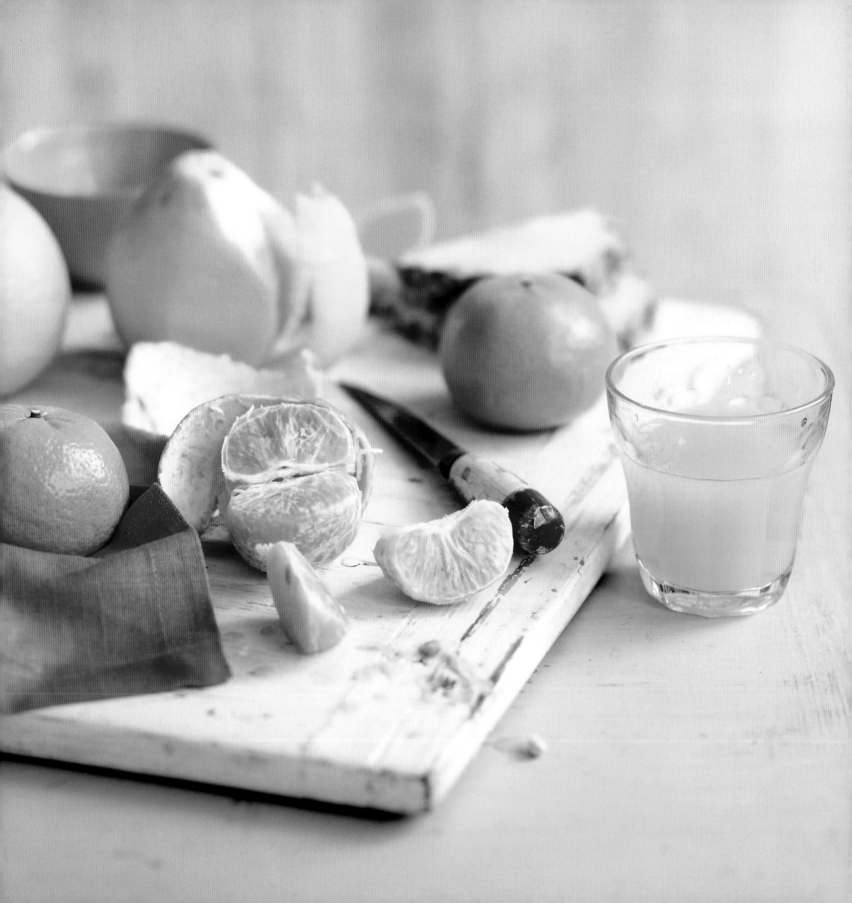

chapter six

Low-FODMAP Diet menu plans

The food plans provided include foods from all food groups and are nutritionally adequate. The Low-FODMAP Diet can provide you with all the nutrients you need each day, because although some foods are excluded, alternatives are included. The meal plan suggestions are in line with the Australian healthy eating guidelines. In general we haven't included quantities because we all have different energy needs, depending on our gender, age, activity level and any medical conditions that may impact on our health. Unless otherwise unsuitable, we suggest you choose low-fat and low-salt options whenever possible. An Accredited Practising Dietitian can provide you with individualised dietary advice and your own food plan.

Note that in all the menu plans, LF means lactose-free.

GENERAL LOW-FODMAP MENU PLAN DAYS 1–7

MEAL	DAY 1 MONDAY	DAY 2 TUESDAY	DAY 3 WEDNESDAY
BREAKFAST	wheat-free cereal lite milk (LF if required) toasted wheat-free bread butter or margarine jam, peanut butter or other suitable spread	poached eggs toasted wheat-free bread butter or margarine jam, peanut butter or other suitable spread	wheat-free cereal lite milk (LF if required) toasted wheat-free bread butter or margarine jam, peanut butter or other suitable spread
LUNCH	rice/corn thins or wheat-free crackers with ham, cheese, lettuce, tomato 1 serve suitable fruit	beef & salad sandwich (wheat-free bread, sliced beef, cheese, sliced tomato, lettuce) 1 serve suitable fruit	Cream of Potato & Parsnip Soup (page 106) wheat-free bread 1 serve suitable fruit
DINNER	Tuscan Tuna Pasta (page 150) salad (capsicum (pepper), baby spinach leaves, celery, chopped herbs) Passionfruit Tart (page 235)	Chinese Chicken on Fried Wild Rice (page 141) sauteed bok choy, celery, carrot, zucchini (courgette) Ice cream (LF if required) 1 serve suitable fruit	Herbed Beef Meatballs with Creamy Potato Nutmeg Mash (page 138) salad (sliced tomato, cucumber, lettuce, celery, capsicum, olives)

DAY 4 THURSDAY	DAY 5 FRIDAY	DAY 6 SATURDAY	DAY 7 SUNDAY

fruit smoothie (bananas or strawberries, yoghurt and lite milk (LF if required))	wheat-free cereal
	lite milk (LF if required)
	toasted wheat-free bread
	butter or margarine
	jam, peanut butter
	    or other suitable spread
		wheat-free cereal
		lite milk (LF if required)
		toasted wheat-free bread
		butter or margarine
		jam, peanut butter
		    or other suitable spread
			lean bacon
			boiled eggs
			grilled tomato
			toasted wheat-free bread
			butter or margarine

Cheese & Herb Polenta
    Wedges (page 127)
1 serve suitable fruit
	Sweet Potato, Blue Cheese
	    & Spinach Frittata
	    (page 113)
	1 serve suitable fruit
		toasted ham & cheese
		    sandwich (wheat-free
		    bread, ham, cheese)
		salad (tomato, lettuce,
		    capsicum (pepper))
		1 serve suitable fruit
			Olive & Eggplant Focaccia
			    (page 185)
			yoghurt (LF if required)
			1 serve suitable fruit

Peppered Lamb with
    Rosemary Cottage
    Potatoes (page 142)
gravy
a suitable green vegetable
an orange vegetable
ice cream (LF if required)
	Balsamic Sesame
	    Swordfish (page 155)
	white rice
	Roast Vegetable Salad
	    (page 123)
	Warm Bananas in Sweet
	    Citrus Sauce (page 224)
		Singapore Noodles
		    (page 174)
		1 cup fruit salad
		    (suitable fruits)
			Roast Pork with
			    Chestnut Stuffing
			    (page 146)
			gravy
			roast potato, sweet potato
			a suitable green vegetable
			New York Cheesecake
			    (page 236)

GENERAL LOW-FODMAP MENU PLAN DAYS 8–14

MEAL	DAY 8 MONDAY	DAY 9 TUESDAY	DAY 10 WEDNESDAY

BREAKFAST	wheat-free cereal
	lite milk (LF if required)
	toasted wheat-free bread
	butter or margarine
	jam, peanut butter
	    or other suitable spread
		poached eggs
		toasted wheat-free bread
		butter or margarine
		jam, peanut butter
		    or other suitable spread
			wheat-free cereal
			lite milk (LF if required)
			toasted wheat-free bread
			butter or margarine
			jam, peanut butter
			    or other suitable spread

LUNCH	beef & salad sandwich
	    (wheat-free bread,
	    sliced beef, sliced
	    tomato, cucumber,
	    lettuce)
	1 serve suitable fruit
		Tuna Lemongrass & Basil
		    Risotto Patties (page 94)
		salad (capsicum (pepper),
		    baby spinach leaves,
		    celery, chopped herbs)
		1 serve suitable fruit
			ham, cheese & salad
			    sandwich (wheat-free
			    bread, ham, cheese,
			    lettuce, grated carrot)
			1 serve suitable fruit

DINNER	Chicken with Maple
	    Mustard Sauce
	    (page 137)
	a suitable green vegetable
	an orange vegetable
	ice cream (LF if required)
		Pork Ragout (page 136)
		cooked gluten-free pasta
			Tomato Chicken Risotto
			    (page 153)
			salad (sliced tomato, celery,
			    lettuce, capsicum (pepper),
			    cucumber)
			ice cream (LF if required)
			½ serve suitable fruit

DAY 11 THURSDAY	DAY 12 FRIDAY	DAY 13 SATURDAY	DAY 14 SUNDAY

wheat-free cereal
lite milk (LF if required)
toasted wheat-free bread
butter or margarine
jam, peanut butter
   or other suitable spread
	omelette with spinach
	   & tomato
	toasted wheat-free bread
	butter or margarine
	jam, peanut butter
	   or other suitable spread
		fruit smoothie
		   (bananas or strawberries,
		   yoghurt and lite milk
		   (LF if required))
			poached eggs
			toasted wheat-free bread
			butter or margarine
			jam, peanut butter
			   or other suitable spread

Lemon Chicken &
   Rice Soup (page 96)
Chilli Capsicum
   Cornbread (page 181)
1 serve suitable fruit
	Roast Vegetable
	   Salad (page 123)
	wheat-free bread
	1 serve suitable fruit
		egg & lettuce sandwich
		   (wheat-free bread,
		   boiled egg, lettuce,
		   mayonnaise)
		1 serve suitable fruit
			Chicken Noodle &
			   Vegetable Soup
			   (page 101)
			wheat-free bread
			1 serve suitable fruit

Chilli Salmon with
   Coriander Salad
   (page 171)
	Lamb & Sweet Potato
	   Curry (page 168)
	steamed rice
		Spinach & Pancetta
		   Pasta (page 160)
		salad (sliced tomato,
		   cucumber, lettuce,
		   capsicum (pepper),
		   celery, olives)
		Dairy-free Baked
		   Rhubarb Custards
		   (page 217)
			French Veal with Herb
			   Rosti (page 164)
			a suitable green vegetable
			an orange vegetable
			Golden Syrup Pudding
			   (page 226)

LACTO-OVO VEGETARIAN LOW-FODMAP 7-DAY MENU PLAN

MEAL	DAY 1 MONDAY	DAY 2 TUESDAY	DAY 3 WEDNESDAY

BREAKFAST	wheat-free cereal
	lite milk (LF if required)
	toasted wheat-free bread
	butter or margarine
	jam, peanut butter
	   or other suitable spread
		poached eggs
		toasted wheat-free bread
		butter or margarine
		jam, peanut butter
		   or other suitable spread
			wheat-free cereal
			lite milk (LF if required)
			toasted wheat-free bread
			butter or margarine
			jam, peanut butter
			   or other suitable spread

LUNCH	rice/corn thins or
	   wheat-free crackers with
	   egg, cheese, tomato,
	   lettuce, mayonnaise
	1 serve suitable fruit
		cheese & salad sandwich
		   (wheat-free bread,
		   cheese, 2 slices tomato,
		   lettuce)
		1 serve suitable fruit
			Cream of Potato
			   & Parsnip Soup
			   (page 106)
			wheat-free bread
			1 serve suitable fruit

DINNER	Thai-inspired Stir-Fry
	   with Tofu & Vermicelli
	   Noodles (omit fish sauce)
	   (page 156)
	Passionfruit Tart
	   (page 235)
		Sweet Potato, Blue Cheese
		   & Spinach Frittata
		   (page 113)
		steamed potato
		a suitable green vegetable
		an orange vegetable
			Fetta, Pumpkin & Chive
			   Fritters (page 102)
			hot chips
			salad (sliced tomato,
			   cucumber, lettuce,
			   capsicum (pepper),
			   celery)
			1 cup fruit salad
			   (suitable fruits)
			ice cream (LF if required)

DAY 4 THURSDAY	DAY 5 FRIDAY	DAY 6 SATURDAY	DAY 7 SUNDAY

wheat-free cereal
lite milk (LF if required)
toasted wheat-free bread
butter or margarine
jam, peanut butter
   or other suitable spread
	omelette with spinach
	   & tomato
	toasted wheat-free bread
	butter or margarine
	jam, peanut butter
	   or other suitable spread
		fruit smoothie (bananas,
		   strawberries, yoghurt and
		   lite milk (LF if required))
			poached eggs
			toasted wheat-free bread
			butter or margarine
			jam, peanut butter
			   or other suitable spread

Cheese & Herb Polenta
   Wedges (page 127)
salad (sliced tomato,
   celery, lettuce, capsicum
   (pepper), cucumber)
1 serve suitable fruit
	Roast Vegetable Salad
	   (page 123)
	wheat-free bread
	1 serve suitable fruit
		toasted tomato &
		   cheese sandwich
		   (wheat-free bread,
		   2 slices tomato,
		   cheese)
		salad (capsicum (pepper),
		   baby spinach leaves,
		   celery, chopped herbs)
			Olive & Eggplant Focaccia
			   (page 185)
			salad (sliced tomato,
			   celery, lettuce, capsicum
			   (pepper), cucumber)
			yoghurt (LF if required)
			1 serve suitable fruit

Tofu, Lemongrass and
   Basil Risotto Patties
   (substitute tofu for
   tuna) (page 94)
sauteed bok choy, celery,
   carrot, zucchini (courgette)
Warm Bananas in
   Sweet Citrus Sauce
   (page 224)
	Zucchini & Potato Torte
	   (omit the bacon)
	   (page 120)
	a suitable green vegetable
	an orange vegetable
		Fetta, Spinach & Pine Nut
		   Crepes (page 132)
		a suitable green vegetable
		an orange vegetable
		ice cream (LF if required)
		1 serve suitable fruit
			Pasta with Ricotta &
			   Lemon (page 160)
			salad (capsicum (pepper),
			   baby spinach leaves,
			   celery, chopped herbs)
			New York Cheesecake
			   (page 236)

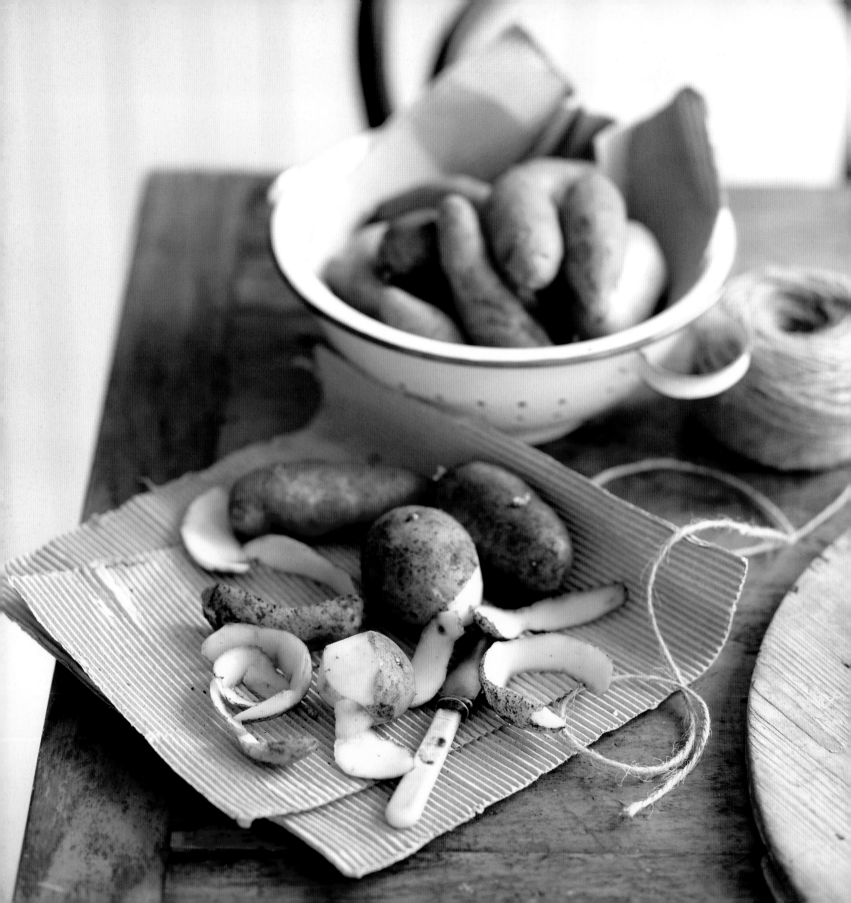

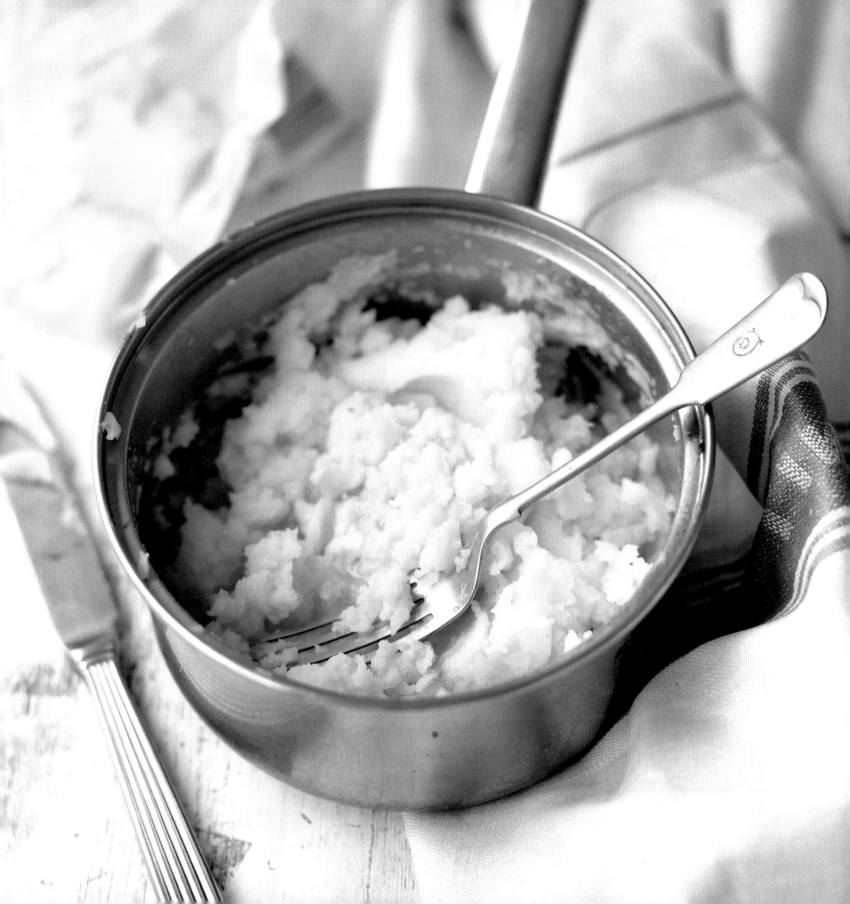

VEGAN LOW-FODMAP 7-DAY MENU PLAN

MEAL	DAY 1 MONDAY	DAY 2 TUESDAY	DAY 3 WEDNESDAY
BREAKFAST	wheat-free high-protein cereal (containing quinoa, amaranth and/or chia) 1–2 tbsp LSA mix soy* or rice milk toasted wheat-free bread milk-free margarine tahini, jam, peanut butter or other suitable spread	wheat-free high-protein cereal (containing quinoa, amaranth and/or chia) 1–2 tbsp LSA mix soy* or rice milk toasted wheat-free bread milk-free margarine tahini, jam, peanut butter or other suitable spread	fruit smoothie (banana or strawberries, soy yoghurt,* soy* or rice milk, chia seeds) toasted wheat-free bread milk-free margarine tahini, jam, peanut butter or other suitable spread
LUNCH	corn/rice thins or wheat-free crackers with tahini, pesto, sliced tomato, lettuce 1 serve suitable fruit	cashew spread sandwich (wheat-free bread, cashew spread, celery, grated carrot, sprinkle of sultanas)	Cheese & Herb Polenta Wedges (use soy cheese) (page 127) 1 serve suitable fruit
DINNER	Thai-inspired Stir-Fry with Tofu & Vermicelli Noodles (omit fish sauce)* (page 156) rice-milk custard	Tempeh* & Sweet Potato Curry (substitute tempeh for lamb) (page 168) white rice non-dairy ice cream	Spiced Tofu* Bites (page 124) rice noodles sauteed bok choy, celery, carrot, zucchini (courgette) non-dairy ice cream 1 cup fruit salad (suitable fruits)

* Soy contains GOS and fructans, however products derived from soy such as milk, yoghurt, cheese, tofu and tempeh do not cause IBS symptoms in most people. You should assess your own tolerance.

DAY 4 THURSDAY	DAY 5 FRIDAY	DAY 6 SATURDAY	DAY 7 SUNDAY
wheat-free high-protein cereal (containing quinoa, amaranth and/or chia) 1–2 tbsp LSA mix soy* or rice milk toasted wheat-free bread milk-free margarine tahini, jam, peanut butter or other suitable spread	wheat-free high-protein cereal (containing quinoa, amaranth and/or chia) 1–2 tbsp LSA mix soy* or rice milk toasted wheat-free bread milk-free margarine tahini, jam, peanut butter or other suitable spread	wheat-free high-protein cereal (containing quinoa, amaranth and/or chia) 1–2 tbsp LSA mix soy* or rice milk toasted wheat-free bread milk-free margarine tahini, jam, peanut butter or other suitable spread	Low-FODMAP Vegan 'sausages'* toasted wheat-free bread milk-free margarine tahini, jam, peanut butter or other suitable spread
Cream of Potato & Parsnip Soup (use rice milk & soy cheese) (page 106) wheat-free bread 1 serve suitable fruit	Roast Vegetable Salad (page 123) wheat-free bread 1 serve suitable fruit	toasted tomato sandwich (wheat-free bread, sliced tomato, baby spinach leaves, wholegrain mustard) 1 serve suitable fruit	Olive & Eggplant Focaccia (omit the cheese) (page 185) handful nuts & seeds 1 serve suitable fruit
Tofu,* Lemongrass and Basil Risotto Patties (substitute tofu for tuna, omit egg) (page 94) salad (capsicum (pepper), baby spinach leaves, celery, chopped herbs) Warm Bananas in Sweet Citrus Sauce (page 224)	Stir-fried Eggplant (aubergine) with Chilli & Coriander (substitute eggplant for kangaroo) (page 158) handful toasted almonds or cashews white rice non-dairy ice cream	Tofu* Kibbeh (substitute tofu* for chicken mince) (page 172) salad (sliced tomato, capsicum (pepper), celery, cucumber, lettuce) non-dairy ice cream	Risotto Milanese (use soy* cheese) (page 154) salad (capsicum (pepper), baby spinach leaves, celery, chopped herbs) Caramel Banana Sago Puddings (use rice milk) (page 224)

LOW-FAT LOW-FODMAP 7-DAY MENU PLAN

MEAL	DAY 1 MONDAY	DAY 2 TUESDAY	DAY 3 WEDNESDAY

BREAKFAST	wheat-free cereal
	skim milk (LF if required)
	toasted wheat-free bread
	jam, marmalade or
	    other low-fat spread
		wheat-free cereal
		skim milk (LF if required)
		toasted wheat-free bread
		jam, marmalade or
		    other low-fat spread
			diet yoghurt (LF if required)
			1 serve suitable fruit
			toasted wheat-free bread
			jam, marmalade or
			    other low-fat spread

LUNCH	rice/corn thins or wheat-free
	    crackers with lean ham,
	    low-fat cheese, sliced
	    tomato, grated carrot,
	    lettuce
	1 serve suitable fruit
		beef & salad sandwich
		    (wheat-free bread,
		    lean sliced beef, low-fat
		    cheese, sliced tomato,
		    lettuce, cucumber)
		1 serve suitable fruit
			Lemon Chicken &
			    Rice Soup (page 96)
			wheat-free bread
			1 serve suitable fruit

DINNER	Tuscan Tuna Pasta
	    (page 150)
	salad (capsicum (pepper),
	    baby spinach leaves,
	    celery, chopped herbs)
	Caramel Banana Sago
	    Puddings (use skim milk)
	    (page 224)
		Chinese Chicken on
		    Fried Wild Rice
		    (page 141)
		steamed bok choy,
		    carrot, zucchini
		    (courgette), celery
		1 serve suitable fruit
		    with jelly
			Herbed Beef Meatballs
			    with Creamy Potato
			    Nutmeg Mash (use skim
			    milk, low-fat cheese &
			    omit butter in the mash)
			    (page 138)
			salad (capsicum (pepper),
			    cucumber, carrot, lettuce)
			low-fat yoghurt (LF if required)

DAY 4 THURSDAY	DAY 5 FRIDAY	DAY 6 SATURDAY	DAY 7 SUNDAY

wheat-free cereal
skim milk (LF if required)
toasted wheat-free bread
jam, marmalade or
    other low-fat spread
	fruit smoothie (strawberry
	    or banana, diet yoghurt,
	    skim milk (LF if required))
		wheat-free cereal
		skim milk (LF if required)
		toasted wheat-free bread
		jam, marmalade or
		    other low-fat spread
			lean bacon
			boiled eggs
			grilled tomato
			toasted wheat-free bread

Crab & Rocket Quinoa
    Salad (page 111)
1 serve suitable fruit
	egg & salad sandwich
	    (wheat-free bread,
	    boiled egg, sliced
	    tomato, sliced cucumber,
	    lettuce)
	1 serve suitable fruit
		toasted ham & cheese
		    sandwich (wheat-free
		    bread, lean ham,
		    low-fat cheese)
		salad (tomato, capsicum
		    (pepper), carrot, celery,
		    lettuce)
		1 serve suitable fruit
			Olive & Eggplant Focaccia
			    (use low-fat cheese)
			    (page 185)
			low-fat yoghurt
			    (LF if required)
			1 serve suitable fruit

Peppered Lamb
    (without the potatoes)
    (page 142)
gravy
mixed roast vegetables
    with rosemary
1 serve suitable fruit
    with jelly
	Balsamic Sesame
	    Swordfish (page 155)
	Roast Vegetable Salad
	    (page 123)
	white rice
	Warm Bananas in Sweet
	    Citrus Sauce (page 224)
		Singapore Noodles
		    (page 174)
		1 serve suitable fruit
		    with jelly
			Roast Pork with Chestnut
			    Stuffing (page 146)
			gravy
			roast potato, sweet potato
			a suitable green vegetable
			Crepes Suzette
			    (use skim milk &
			    low-fat margarine)
			    (page 223)

DAIRY-FREE LOW-FODMAP 7-DAY MENU PLAN*

MEAL	DAY 1 MONDAY	DAY 2 TUESDAY	DAY 3 WEDNESDAY

BREAKFAST	wheat-free cereal
	rice milk
	toasted wheat-free bread
	milk-free margarine
	jam, peanut butter
	   or other suitable spread
		wheat-free cereal
		rice milk
		toasted wheat-free bread
		milk-free margarine
		jam, peanut butter
		   or other suitable spread
			poached eggs
			milk-free margarine
			jam, peanut butter
			   or other suitable spread

LUNCH	ham & salad sandwich
	   (wheat-free bread,
	   ham, sliced tomato,
	   cucumber, lettuce)
	1 serve suitable fruit
		beef & salad sandwich
		   (wheat-free bread,
		   sliced beef, sliced
		   tomato, baby spinach
		   leaves, grated carrot)
		1 serve suitable fruit
			Lemon Chicken &
			   Rice Soup (page 96)
			Chilli Capsicum
			   Cornbread (page 181)
			1 serve suitable fruit

DINNER	Tuscan Tuna Pasta
	   (page 150)
	salad (capsicum, baby
	   spinach leaves, celery,
	   chopped herbs)
	Caramel Banana Sago
	   Puddings (use rice milk)
	   (page 224)
		Chinese Chicken on
		   Fried Wild Rice
		   (page 141)
		sauteed bok choy, celery,
		   carrot, zucchini
		non-dairy ice cream
		1 cup fruit salad
		   (suitable fruits)
			Goat's Cheese & Chive
			   Souffles (page 118)
			hot chips
			salad (sliced tomato,
			   celery, cucumber,
			   carrot, lettuce)
			non-dairy ice cream

* A dairy-free diet is different from a lactose-free diet. Although non-dairy sources of goat and sheep milk still contain lactose, many people choose to follow a dairy-free diet. For this reason, we have provided a sample menu plan.

DAY 4 THURSDAY	DAY 5 FRIDAY	DAY 6 SATURDAY	DAY 7 SUNDAY
wheat-free cereal	fruit smoothie (banana or	omelette with spinach	poached eggs
rice milk	strawberries, non-dairy	and tomato	milk-free margarine
toasted wheat-free bread	yoghurt, non-dairy milk	toasted wheat-free bread	jam, peanut butter
milk-free margarine	(LF if required))	milk-free margarine	or other suitable spread
jam, peanut butter	toasted wheat-free bread	jam, peanut butter	
or other suitable spread	milk-free margarine	or other suitable spread	
	jam, peanut butter		
	or other suitable spread		
Tuna Lemongrass & Basil	Roast Vegetable Salad	toasted ham, sandwich	Olive & Eggplant Focaccia
Risotto Patties (page 94)	(page 123)	(wheat-free bread, ham,	(use pecorino cheese)
salad (capsicum (pepper),	wheat-free bread	2 slices tomato, baby	(page 185)
baby spinach leaves,	1 serve suitable fruit	spinach leaves, goat's	1 serve suitable fruit
celery, chopped herbs)		cheese, grainy mustard)	
1 serve suitable fruit		1 serve suitable fruit	
Lamb & Sweet Potato	Balsamic Sesame Swordfish	Singapore Noodles	French Veal with Herb
Curry (page 168)	(page 155)	(page 174)	Rosti (page 164)
steamed rice	white rice	Dairy-free Baked Rhubarb	a suitable green vegetable
	a suitable green vegetable	Custards (page 217)	an orange vegetable
	an orange vegetable		Polenta Dessert Cake
	Warm Bananas in Sweet		with Lime & Strawberry
	Citrus Sauce (page 224)		Syrup (substitute
			dairy-free margarine
			for butter) (page 238)

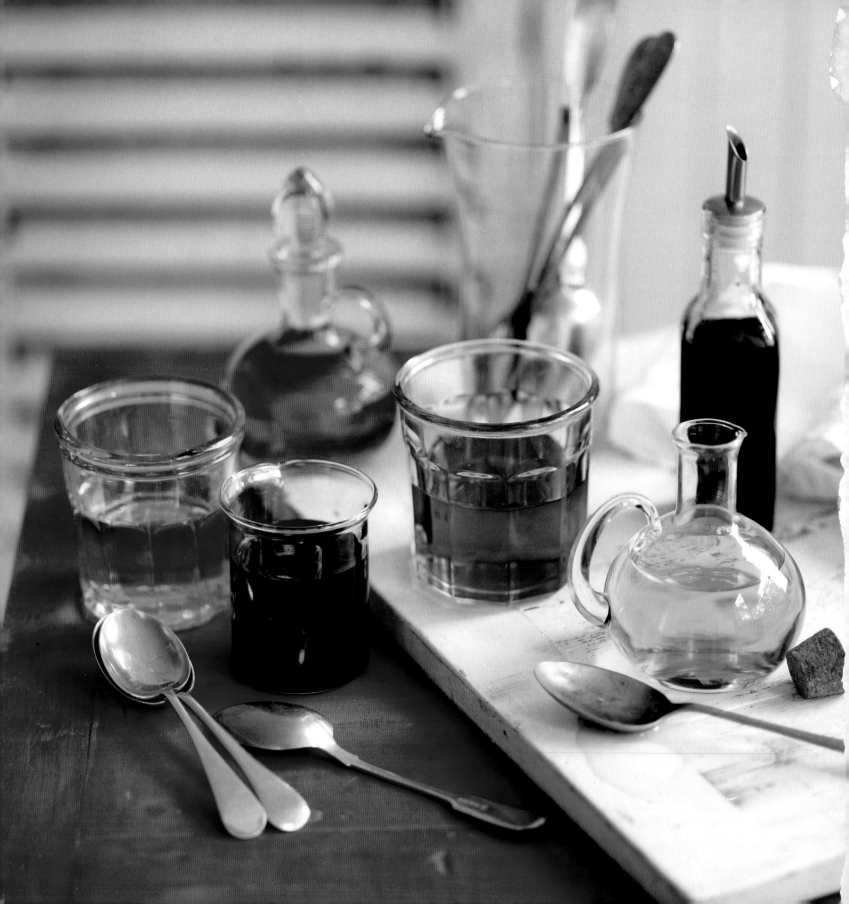

chapter seven

Making the Low-FODMAP Diet easier

Flavouring food

The Low-FODMAP Diet means changing your cooking methods and what you stock in your pantry. For instance, many people find they miss the flavour of onion in their cooking. But you can boost the flavours of your dishes by using the following Low-FODMAP herbs and spices: allspice, asafoetida, basil, bay leaves, caraway, cardamom, cayenne pepper, celery seeds, chervil, chilli, chives, cinnamon, cloves, coriander, cumin, curry leaves, dill seeds, elderflower, fenugreek, galangal, ginger, juniper berries, kaffir lime leaves, lavender, lemon basil, lemongrass, lemon myrtle, lemon thyme, licorice, mace, marjoram, mustard, nutmeg, oregano, paprika, parsley, pepper, peppermint, poppy seeds, rosemary, saffron, sage, sesame seeds, spearmint, star anise, sumac, Szechuan pepper, vanilla.

Some people with IBS do not tolerate spicy foods, so use the spices according to your own preferences and tolerance.

GARLIC-FLAVOURED OIL

Some IBS sufferers can tolerate a small amount of garlic; others cannot. Garlic-flavoured oil provides a good flavour substitute. The simplest way to do this when using oil to cook is to place a couple of peeled garlic cloves in the heating oil, brown lightly, then discard the cloves before adding the other ingredients.

There is a wide range of commercially prepared garlic-infused oils available. If preparing at home, strict instructions need to be followed; fresh garlic, like many other vegetables and herbs when preserved in oil, can be a breeding ground for Clostridium botulinum, the organism that causes botulism. To make garlic-infused oil for cooking, use four to five peeled cloves of commercially treated (sanitised) garlic; this means garlic that comes from the supermarket as opposed to home-grown or organic garlic (the botulism arises from traces of soil). Put the garlic in a jar with 125 ml olive, canola or peanut oil. Refrigerate immediately and keep for no more than seven days. If you are planning on using your home-prepared infused oil as part of a salad dressing, you can acidify the garlic before immersing it in oil, which will allow you to keep it longer – two to three weeks. To do this, place four to five peeled cloves of sanitised garlic in a jar and douse with an equal amount of vinegar (for 40 g garlic use 40 ml vinegar) then add 125 ml olive, canola or peanut oil. Keep refrigerated during the entire storage period and use within the suggested time. When making the dressing, discard the garlic and adjust the amount of vinegar to taste. For a quick solution, rub your salad bowl with a cut clove of garlic – organic or fresh from the garden is fine – before adding the other ingredients.

Reading food labels

Always read the label to see if a certain food is suitably low in FODMAPs. Ingredients are given in descending order of ingoing weight (ie, the greatest amount is listed first). FODMAPs are only a problem when consumed regularly and in significant amounts. If a food contains more than tiny amounts, you should avoid it. Some foods, however, may contain FODMAP ingredients in too small a quantity to cause gut symptoms, and so can still be eaten. For example, if honey is less than 5 per cent of the whole product it will probably be suitable to consume. See also the table opposite.

AVOIDING ONION AND GARLIC

The one exception to the rule that small amounts of FODMAP ingredients are suitable to eat is *onion*. We recommend you avoid *all* foods containing onion, even if it is present in minute amounts. Since onion is one of the major triggers of IBS symptoms, it is important to be on the 'onion lookout'

LOW-FODMAP FOODS FOR YOUR PANTRY AND FRIDGE

INGREDIENT TYPE	INGREDIENT	WHERE TO BUY
flours – essential	cornflour (cornstarch) – must be made from maize (corn)	supermarkets
	potato flour	supermarkets and Asian grocery shops
	rice flour (preferably fine rice flour)	supermarkets and Asian grocery shops
	soy flour (debittered)*	health-food shops and online stores
	tapioca flour	supermarkets and Asian grocery shops
flours – worthwhile	amaranth flour	health-food shops and online stores
	arrowroot	supermarkets
	buckwheat flour (be aware that some are blends and contain wheat flour)	health-food shops and online stores
	chickpea/besan flour* (an alternative to soy)	health-food shops and Indian grocery shops
	millet flour	health-food shops and online stores
	quinoa flour (pronounced 'keen-wah')	health-food shops
oils	cooking oil (e.g. canola oil, olive oil, rice bran oil), olive oil spray	supermarkets
sauces and dressings	fish sauce, hoisin sauce, oyster sauce, soy sauce, sweet chilli sauce, tomato sauce, mayonnaise, pesto, balsamic vinegar, white vinegar	supermarkets
others	almond meal, cocoa powder, pine nuts, polenta, vanilla essence, wheat-free breadcrumbs	supermarkets
	xanthan gum	health-food shops
herbs and spices	see flavouring food information, opposite	

* These contain GOS and fructans, but in small amounts as part of a recipe, do not cause IBS symptoms in most people. You should assess your own tolerance.

when purchasing packaged foods such as stocks, gravies, soups, sauces, marinades, potato crisps and other savoury snacks such as rice crackers. Onion is not an allergen, so it does not have to be declared on the ingredients list if it is a component of other ingredients. This means that onion could be 'hiding' in such ingredients as chicken salt, vegetable salt, vegetable powder and dehydrated vegetables. These ingredients can also contain hidden garlic, so we recommend that you read the ingredients lists on packaged foods and avoid anything that contains these ingredients, as well as onion, onion powder and golden shallots.

To avoid onion in your meals, look for onion and 'hidden' onion ingredients in freshly cooked food and packaged food items, and do not use onion in your own cooking. You should avoid brown, white or red onion, golden shallots, leeks and the white part of spring onions in all your cooking. Alternatives to onion include chives, the green part of spring onion (although you should test your own tolerance here), fresh and dried herbs and spices, and asafoetida powder, a spice that tastes similar to onion and is available in Indian spice shops.

WHEN SHOULD WHEAT BE AVOIDED?

Wheat is only a problem ingredient when consumed in large amounts, such as in breads, cereals or pasta (see the list on page 41). Foods that contain minimal amounts of wheat, such as soy sauce, will not typically be a problem for people following the Low-FODMAP Diet.

The Australian food labelling laws make it compulsory for manufacturers to declare all wheat-derived ingredients but it is important to realise that many wheat ingredients are actually chains of glucose and do not contain fructans, and so are safe on the Low-FODMAP Diet. These include wheat starch, wheat thickeners, wheat maltodextrin, wheat dextrin, wheat dextrose, wheat glucose and wheat colour caramel.

INTERPRETING FOOD LABELS

Here are two examples of how food labels should be interpreted, both with fructose as the FODMAP ingredient.

A PINEAPPLE-FLAVOURED SPORTS DRINK

The ingredients list reads: 'Distilled water, *fructose*, reconstituted fruit juices (pineapple, grape), food acid, flavour, preservative'. Since fructose is the second ingredient in this sports drink, fructose is present in large amounts and is the main sweetener of the product. We would therefore recommend that you avoid consuming this product.

A WHEAT-FREE BREAD MIX

The ingredients list reads: 'Maize flour, potato flour, tapioca flour, milk solids, bicarbonate of soda, salt, *fructose*, preservative'. Since fructose is the seventh (and second-last) ingredient in this bread mix, it is present as an incidental ingredient only (less than salt) and does not act as a sweetener in the product. It would be acceptable to consume this product, even though fructose is an ingredient.

For more information on how to read food labels, see this book's website, foodintolerancemanagementplan.com.au.

WHEAT-FREE VERSUS GLUTEN-FREE FOODS

A Low-FODMAP Diet is *not* a gluten-free diet. Gluten-free foods do not contain wheat, rye, oats or barley, and so can often be suitable for people on the Low-FODMAP Diet. People following the Low-FODMAP Diet can, however, still include barley and oats and usually small amounts of wheat, and some people can also tolerate small amounts of rye.

It is important to note that many gluten-free foods contain FODMAPs. Examples include fruits, such as apples and pears, and legumes, such as baked beans.

There are other clear differences between Low-FODMAP and gluten-free diets, such as the following:

1. *The diets are treating different underlying problems.* People with coeliac disease suffer inflammation in and injury to the small intestine. It is a condition that can lead to serious medical problems if not diagnosed and treated with a strict gluten-free diet for life. IBS, on the other hand, is not associated with injury to the bowel. So, while it causes lots of symptoms and can make life miserable if the Low-FODMAP Diet is not strictly followed, it does not have serious medical consequences.

2. *One requires absolute restriction and the other only a reduced dose.* People with coeliac disease *must* remove absolutely *all* gluten from their diet so that their intestine heals and remains healed. With the Low-FODMAP Diet, however, it is all about dose – a small amount of FODMAPs are okay but larger amounts can cause symptoms.

3. *The consequences of breaking the diet are vastly different.* When someone with coeliac disease consumes gluten, they often experience gut and other symptoms, such as a 'foggy head', and even a flare-up of gut inflammation with a slow recovery. When someone on the Low-FODMAP Diet consumes large amounts of FODMAPs, they will also experience many symptoms, but these will resolve once the FODMAPs have left the gut, and there will be no ongoing consequences.

4. *One allows flexibility and the other none.* A gluten-free diet is a very strict diet; people with coeliac disease who stray from it suffer badly. The Low-FODMAP Diet is not as strict and, once you know your own tolerances, has much room for flexibility.

The low-FODMAP Diet is therefore very different from the gluten-free diet and the two should never be confused. Although they have the common element of avoiding wheat, the Low-FODMAP Diet restricts the carbohydrate (fructan) content of wheat, whereas the focus of a gluten-free diet is to avoid the protein (gluten) content of wheat completely.

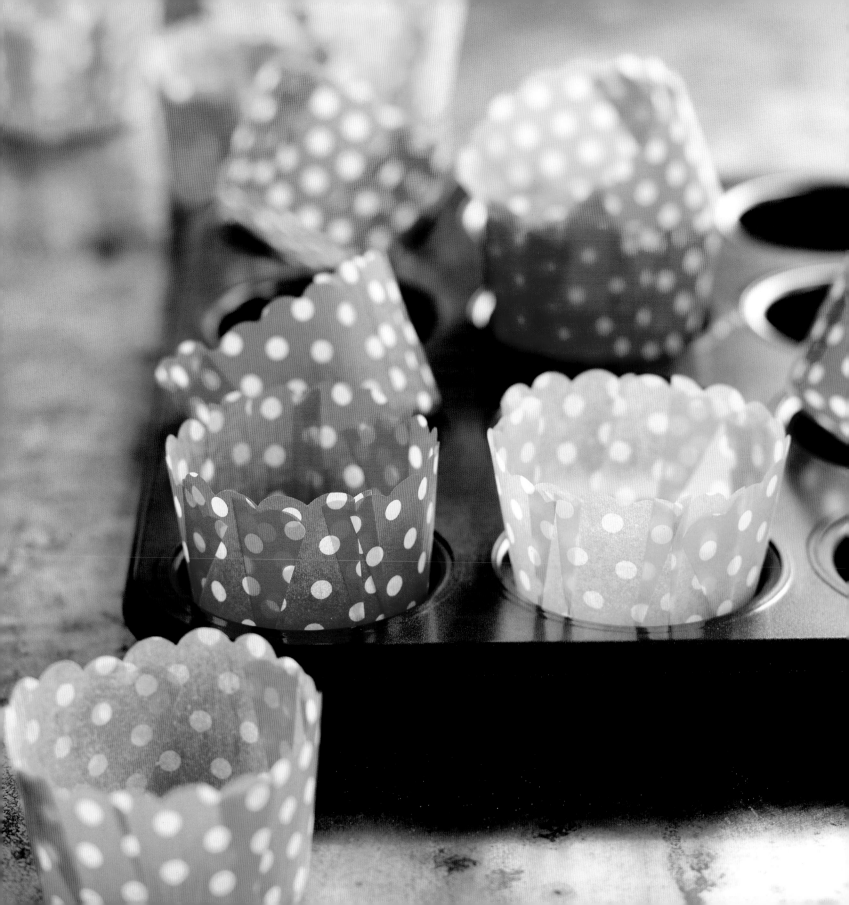

chapter eight
Special occasions and the Low-FODMAP Diet

Entertaining at home

MENU IDEAS FOR DINNER PARTIES

Inexpensive

Lemon Chicken & Rice Soup (page 96)

Zucchini & Potato Torte (page 120)

steamed seasonal vegetables

Caramel Banana Sago Puddings (page 224)

Fancy

Goat's Cheese & Chive Souffle (page 118)

French Veal with Herb Rosti (page 164)

steamed baby carrots and wilted spinach

Cinnamon Chilli Chocolate Brulees (page 215)

Easy

Lemon Oregano Chicken Legs (page 96)

Chilli Salmon with Coriander Salad (page 171)

Baked Ricotta with Stewed Spiced Rhubarb (page 232)

Seafood

Tuna, Lemongrass & Basil Risotto Patties (page 94)

Dukka-crusted Trevalla (page 150)

Creamy Potato Nutmeg Mash (page 138)

steamed seasonal green vegetables

Crepes Suzette (page 223)

Summer

Sweet Potato, Blue Cheese & Spinach Frittata (page 113)

Balsamic Sesame Swordfish (page 155)

Mixed Potato Salad with Bacon & Herb Dressing (page 99)

Garden Salad (page 166)

Passionfruit Tart (page 235)

Asian

Pork & Crunchy Noodle Salad (page 114)

Chinese Chicken on Fried Wild Rice (page 141)

Warm Bananas in Sweet Citrus Sauce (page 224)

Italian

Olive & Eggplant Focaccia (page 185)

Spinach & Pancetta Pasta (page 160)

Panna Cotta with Rosewater Cinnamon Syrup (page 218)

Vegetarian

Spiced Tofu Bites (page 124)

Thai-inspired Stir Fry (omit fish sauce) (page 156)

steamed jasmine rice

Polenta Dessert Cake with Lime & Strawberry Syrup (page 238)

Dairy-free

Goat's Cheese & Chive Souffle (page 118)

Chicken with Maple Mustard Sauce (page 137)

Roast Vegetable Salad (page 123)

Dairy-free Baked Rhubarb Custards (page 217)

Low-fat

Crab & Rocket Quinoa Salad (page 111)

Prosciutto Chicken with Sage Polenta (page 130)

steamed seasonal vegetables

Sweet Chestnut Cake (use low fat-yoghurt, page 208)

Winter

Cream of Potato & Parsnip Soup (page 106)

Lamb & Sweet Potato Curry (page 168)

steamed jasmine rice

Gooey Chocolate Puddings (page 212)

SUGGESTIONS FOR FINGER FOOD AND PICNICS

Food that is suitable for a cocktail party as finger food is often also good for picnics and lunchboxes.

- Tuna, Lemongrass & Basil Risotto Patties (page 94)

- Lemon Oregano Chicken Legs (page 96)

- Zucchini & Potato Torte (cut into bite-sized pieces for finger food, page 120)

- Fetta, Pumpkin & Chive Fritters (page 102)

- Sweet Potato, Blue Cheese & Spinach Frittata (cut into bite-sized pieces for finger food, page 113)

- Chicken Tikka Skewers (page 124)

- Pumpkin, Rice and Ricotta Slice (cut into bite-sized pieces for finger food, page 117)

- Cheese & Herb Polenta Wedges (page 127)

- Sultana Scones (page 188)

- Lemon Lime Slice (page 199)

- Lemon Friands (page 201)

For finger food you could also try:

- Sausage Rolls (page 104)

- Spiced Tofu Bites (page 124)

- Mocha Mud Cake (page 192)

- Moist Banana Cake (page 207)

- Strawberry Slice (page 230)

- Sweet Chestnut Cake (page 208)

And for picnics or lunchboxes you could also try:

- Mixed Potato Salad with Bacon & Herb Dressing (page 99)

- Chicken Salad with Herb Dressing (page 107)

- Gluten-free Fatoush Salad with Chicken (page 108)

- Crab & Rocket Quinoa Salad (page 111)

- Egg & Spinach Salad (page 121)

- Roast Vegetable Salad (page 123)

- Pork & Crunchy Noodle Salad (page 114)

- Spiced Tofu Bites (page 124)

- Seed & Spice Muffins (page 203)

- Macaroons (page 186)

- Pineapple Muffins (page 205)

Eating out

As time passes, you will become very familiar and quite confident in following the Low-FODMAP Diet at home. You should enjoy the same confidence in restaurants and cafes. Eating at a restaurant should be an enjoyable social experience, so here are some tips for eliminating the stress and cranking up the fun.

If you experience severe symptoms after a small 'breakout' from the diet, you'll know to be more strict next time. If, however, you can enjoy a brief deviation from the strict Low-FODMAP Diet without suffering too many symptoms, then you might choose to be a little less strict when eating out.

LOOK FOR FRIENDLY PLACES TO DINE

If you are new to the Low-FODMAP Diet, look for establishments that demonstrate an awareness of gluten-free eating and indicate on the menu which options are wheat-free. The waiters in such eateries usually have an understanding of food intolerances and may be more likely to oblige your special requests. Although a Low-FODMAP Diet is *not* a gluten-free diet, they both restrict wheat. Restaurants and cafes that offer gluten-free options will more likely offer you a more extensive menu.

Some of these establishments offer a dedicated gluten-free menu, others identify gluten-free menu items within the usual menu, and still others state on the menu that they will modify dishes to make them gluten-free. For websites listing 'gluten-free friendly' restaurants, visit this book's own website, foodintolerancemanagementplan.com.au.

TELEPHONE AHEAD

If the restaurant or cafe does not specifically advertise gluten-free or wheat-free meals, it is always a good idea to phone in advance and explain your special dietary needs to the chef. Chefs are becoming increasingly aware of food intolerances. Even if they don't recognise names like 'the Low-FODMAP Diet' or 'fructose malabsorption', you can still explain your special dietary needs so that they understand your requirements. Tell them what you can and can't eat. Ask about the ingredients in specific dishes. Give them enough information to help you – without information overload. You could even send a list of foods to the restaurant. This may feel daunting at first, but confidence builds with practice. The chef may be able to advise which meals would be suitable for you or even prepare you a special dish. Reiterate your requirements when you arrive at the restaurant, to ensure the meal that arrives is low in FODMAPs.

The following points might help you enjoy a low-FODMAP dining experience, but use them as a guide only rather than all at once! Ask as many questions as you need to feel confident that your meal is low in FODMAPs.

- Write a summary of your Low-FODMAP Diet on a business-card-sized menu card and carry it in your wallet to use when explaining your dietary needs. A dietitian could help you with this.

- A 'gluten-free meal with no onion' is a simplified description of the Low-FODMAP Diet that is easy for waiters and chefs to understand.

- Small amounts of wheat can generally be tolerated by IBS sufferers – you do not need to avoid every crumb on the Low-FODMAP Diet. This means that you need not religiously avoid breadcrumbs on vegetables or a schnitzel, or croutons in salads. If you do wish to avoid even these small amounts of wheat, ask for your meal to be prepared without them, or just leave them on the side of your plate.

- Wheat as an ingredient in sauces (such as soy sauce, teriyaki sauce, malt vinegar or mayonnaise) is not a problem for the Low-FODMAP Diet.

- Hidden sources of onion can include stock (used in risottos and soups), gravy, dressings, relishes and sauces. It may also have been used in marinades for meat and chicken. Sausages often contain onion. Ask for gravies and sauces to be served separately.

- Stuffing in a roast or barbecue chicken contains breadcrumbs and usually onion, so it is usually best to avoid the stuffing. Also check the seasoning on top, which could contain onion powder.

- If you break your diet by eating a FODMAP intentionally or unintentionally, you may suffer IBS symptoms, but a break in the diet will not cause any gastrointestinal damage, so your symptom control is entirely up to you.

- Some cuisines, such as Japanese, are friendlier than others. The following table lists meals from different cuisines that are often low in FODMAPs, or will require little modification to become so.

LOW-FODMAP SELECTIONS FROM DIFFERENT CUISINES

CUISINE	LIKELY LOW-FODMAP DISHES
Middle Eastern and Indian	kebabs (skewered meat); tikka dishes (yoghurt marinade); tandoori dishes; steamed rice; kheer (rice pudding – note contains milk and often pistachios); kulfi (Indian ice cream – note contains milk and often pistachios)
South-East Asian	fried rice (check there is no spring onion); steamed or sticky rice; rice paper rolls; sushi (check fillings); omelettes (check fillings); steamed fish; chilli, ginger or peppered prawns, meat, fish or poultry; roast duck or pork; steamed and stir-fried vegetables; rice noodle soup; stir-fries (request no onion or spring onion and check sauces); sweet sticky rice; sorbets (check flavours)
Italian	risotto (ask for no onion and check for onion-free stock); gluten-free pasta with pesto, carbonara or many marinara sauces; steamed mussels; grilled chicken breast or veal steak; shrimp cocktail; mozzarella tomato salad; antipasto (no artichokes); polenta; steamed vegetables; gelato (check flavours); granita; zabaglione (custard – note contains lactose)
Mexican	plain corn chips with chilli cheese dip (chile con queso); tacos (beef or chicken with shredded lettuce, cheese, cucumber and sour cream filling); tamales (stuffed cornmeal – check no onion); tostadas (filled fried corn tortillas – choose beef or chicken filling with no onion); fajitas (no onion, ask for maize tortilla); nachos (no salsa, no refried beans, no guacamole); arroz (rice); arroz con leche (rice pudding – note contains milk); flan (custard); helados (ice cream, sherbert or sorbet – check flavours)
Pub food	plain grills or roasts with vegetables (check gravy, suitable vegetables); grilled fish; risotto (check for onion-free stock and suitable vegetables); salads (check dressings, no onion); flourless cakes; sorbets; meringues

TAKE YOUR OWN

You may also like to:

- Take your own wheat-free bread or roll to a sandwich bar and ask them to fill it with your favourite low-FODMAP fillings.

- Take your wheat-free bread or bread roll to a hamburger restaurant where they can provide an onion-free meat patty and fillings.

- Take your own gluten-free pasta to a restaurant (check before you leave home) and ask them to top it with a low-FODMAP sauce.

- Take your own pizza base to a restaurant and ask them to top it with onion-free sauces and low-FODMAP ingredients.

ENJOY YOURSELF!

When your low-FODMAP meal arrives, enjoy it! Relax and appreciate the pleasures of eating out. Afterwards, it is kind to provide feedback to the restaurant staff about your dining experience. If you've had a positive experience, you could recommend the venue to your friends and family, and let websites and other restaurant-awareness programs know of your good experience.

Eating at friends' houses

Much of the advice given already is appropriate for friends and family. Why not lend them this book to read, so they can fully understand why you follow a special diet, and what the Low-FODMAP Diet is all about? Encourage your friends and relatives to read food labels, so they are aware not only of problem foods, but also those that are suitable. If they cook regularly for you, you may wish to provide them with a copy of Sue's *Low-FODMAP Shopping Guide*. Encourage them to ask questions – the more people understand your dietary needs, the better it will be for you.

It's best not to assume that your friends and family can cater for your Low-FODMAP Diet. They may forget or make mistakes, not because they don't care, but just because they are only human. To lessen the stress for you and your hosts, here are some useful suggestions:

- *Ask politely what they intend to serve* – then decide if you'd like to ask them to make alterations, or if you would rather self-cater. Discreetly taking your own food will help ensure you don't end up starving all night, and can enjoy food with the others.

- *If necessary, eat before you go* – especially if you know in advance that the menu will not be suitable. Then you can just top up on suitable snacks during the event. Don't let the food (or lack of it) spoil your good time or anyone else's.

Travelling

Although you have special dietary needs, this should not prevent you from enjoying your travel experiences. The key to a successful holiday is planning, planning, planning!

Airline travel can be difficult, but airline companies are increasingly aware of special dietary needs, and the chances are you will be able to organise a suitable meal. Here are some helpful travel suggestions to ensure you keep your IBS symptoms to a minimum, your tastebuds satisfied and your stomach full:

- Airlines differ in the service they provide – you may need to choose the airline based specifically on the food service it offers.

- Notify the airline of your special dietary need when you book. Do not rely on your travel agent to advise the airline of your special dietary need – you should contact the airline yourself.

- Confirm with your airline a few days before travelling that your special dietary need has been recorded, and check again when you collect your ticket for departure.

- Carry safe snacks with you just in case there is a problem with your meal.

- You may like to take some phrases explaining your dietary needs in the languages of the countries you'll be travelling in. Visit this book's website, foodintolerancemanagementplan.com.au, for a list of translations.

TIPS FOR TRAVEL WITHIN AUSTRALIA

Your mode of travel, the time it takes to get there and the style of accommodation when you arrive are just some of the things you'll need to consider before you leave.

It goes without saying that you are likely to have greater access to specialty foods in larger cities. More remote holiday locations will require a bit more planning on your part, as specialty breads, pasta, biscuits and snack foods will vary in availability. We recommend that you take non-perishable packet foods, such as breakfast cereal, dry biscuits and snacks, with you. Staple safe foods such as unprocessed meat, fish, chicken, fruits, vegetables, nuts, seeds, rice, potato, milk (though not always lactose-free) and cheese should be available at most destinations.

If you have booked a package tour that includes catering, you must organise your special meals *before* you go – it will be quite difficult for the company to arrange a meal for you once you have departed. That way you'll be able to enjoy your meal and not be restricted to boiled rice, steamed vegetables and grilled chicken every night.

TIPS FOR OVERSEAS TRAVEL

If you carry specialty foods, such as gluten-free biscuits or cereal, with you in your luggage, then you must declare it to customs in most countries. It is advisable to take a letter with you from your doctor stating you have a condition that requires special food. It may also be advisable to contact Australian Customs regarding food restrictions in other countries.

Awareness of specialty dietary requirements varies around the world. In the United Kingdom, Ireland, Italy and Germany, for example, gluten-free products are relatively easy to purchase. In some other European countries, however, especially in Eastern Europe, and across the Middle East, it can be difficult to find wheat-free food products. In many Asian countries, much of the local food is rice- tapioca- or potato-based, so it is less challenging to find wheat-free food.

When eating in restaurants overseas, do not assume that the items on the menu are the same as those at home. If possible, find out the ingredients in each item. Language barriers can often pose a problem – visit this book's website, foodintolerancemanagementplan.com.au, for a list of useful translations and print them out to take with you.

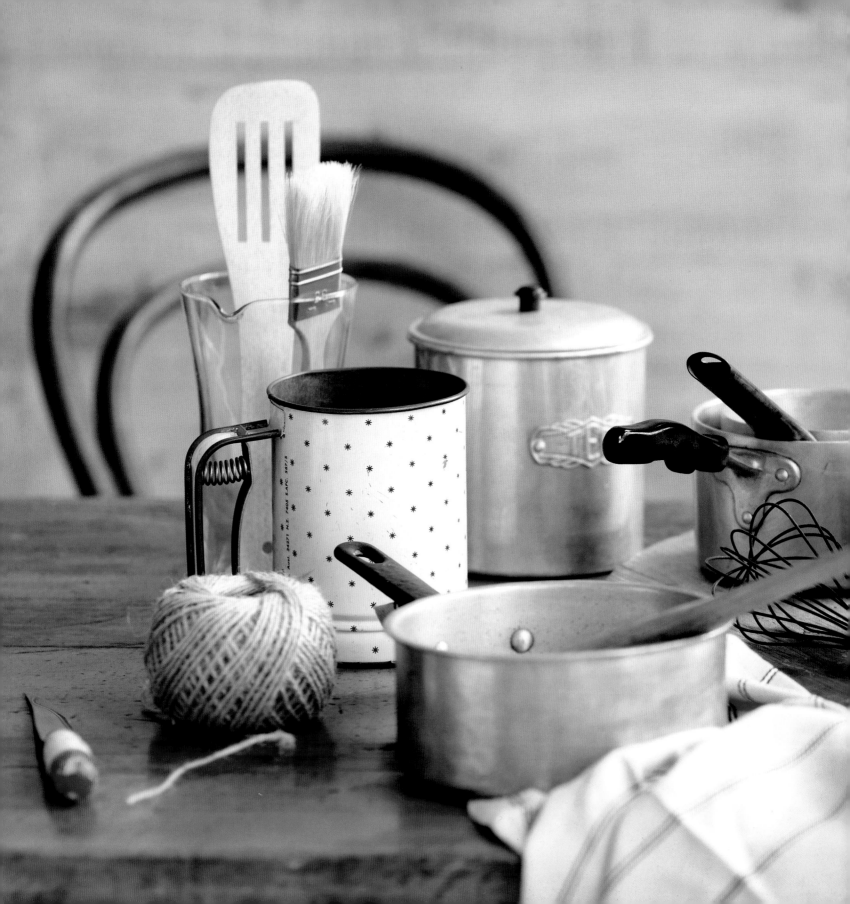

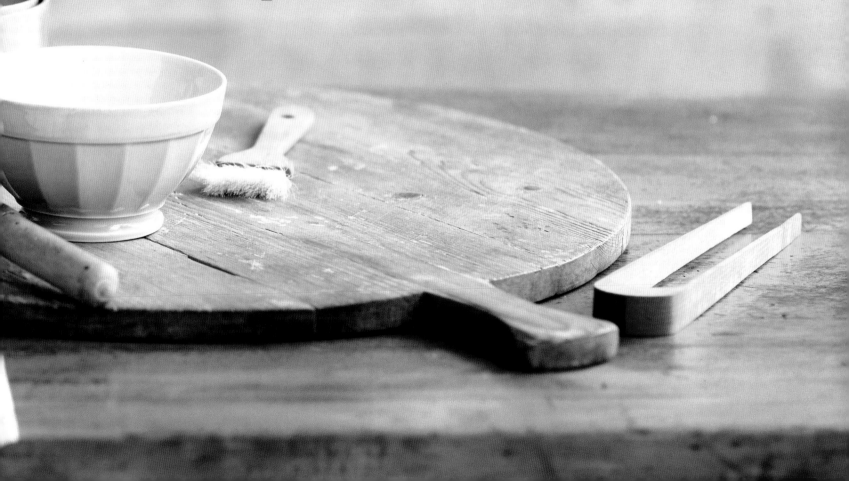

Part Two
Low-FODMAP recipes

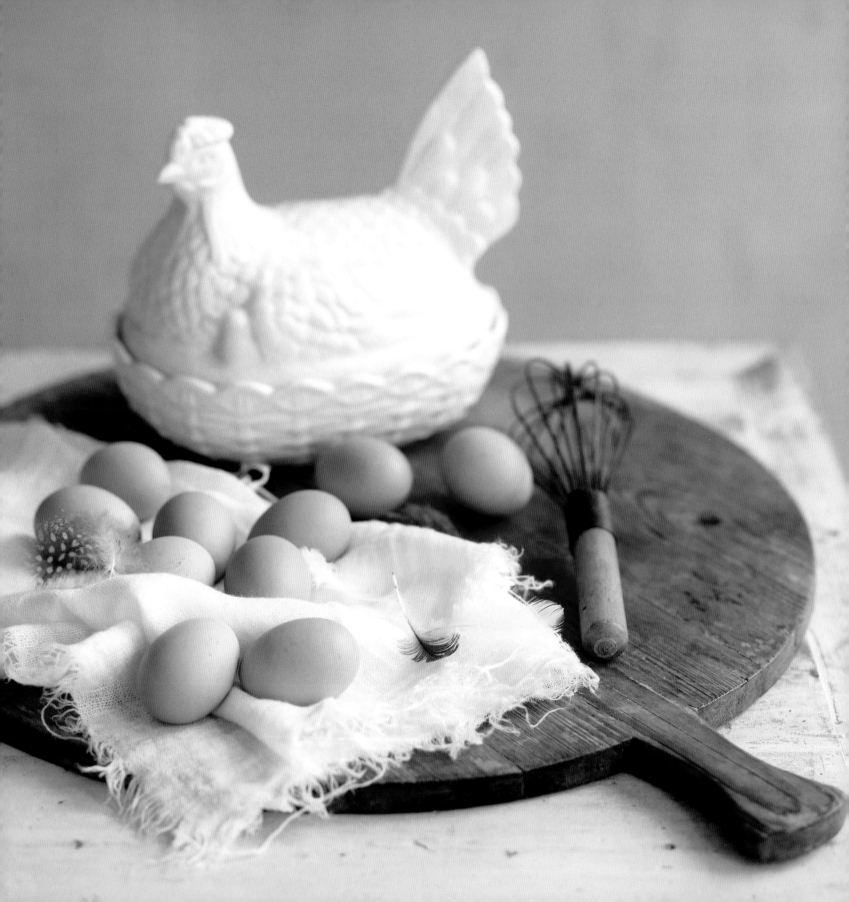

Light meals

Tuna, lemongrass and basil risotto patties

SERVES 4

These flavoursome patties are delicious as a main meal with a salad on the side, but they are also great to have as a quick lunch – very transportable and very tasty!

Pour the stock into a large saucepan and bring to the boil. Add the rice and cook for 10–12 minutes or until tender. Drain any excess liquid. While still warm, stir in the tuna, lemongrass and basil and mix until well combined. Transfer to a medium bowl and set aside to cool to room temperature.

Preheat the oven to 150°C.

Stir the beaten egg and ⅓ cup (40 g) breadcrumbs into the cooled rice and season with salt and pepper. Form the mixture into eight large balls, then flatten to make patties. (If the mixture is not quite firm enough, add more breadcrumbs.)

Place the cornflour, extra egg and remaining breadcrumbs in three small bowls. Toss the patties in the cornflour, then in the beaten egg, and finally in the breadcrumbs. Set aside on a plate.

Heat a little oil in a medium frying pan over medium–high heat. Add four patties to the pan and cook for 2–3 minutes or until evenly browned on both sides. Transfer to a baking tray and keep warm in the oven. Heat a little more oil in the pan and cook the remaining patties. Serve warm with salad.

3 cups (750 ml) onion-free chicken stock (gluten-free if following a gluten-free diet)

¾ cup (150 g) arborio rice

110 g tinned tuna in oil, drained

2 tablespoons finely chopped lemongrass

2 tablespoons chopped basil

1 egg, lightly beaten

1⅓ cups (160 g) gluten-free breadcrumbs

salt and freshly ground black pepper

½ cup (75 g) maize cornflour

1 egg, extra, lightly beaten

canola oil, for pan-frying

garden salad, to serve

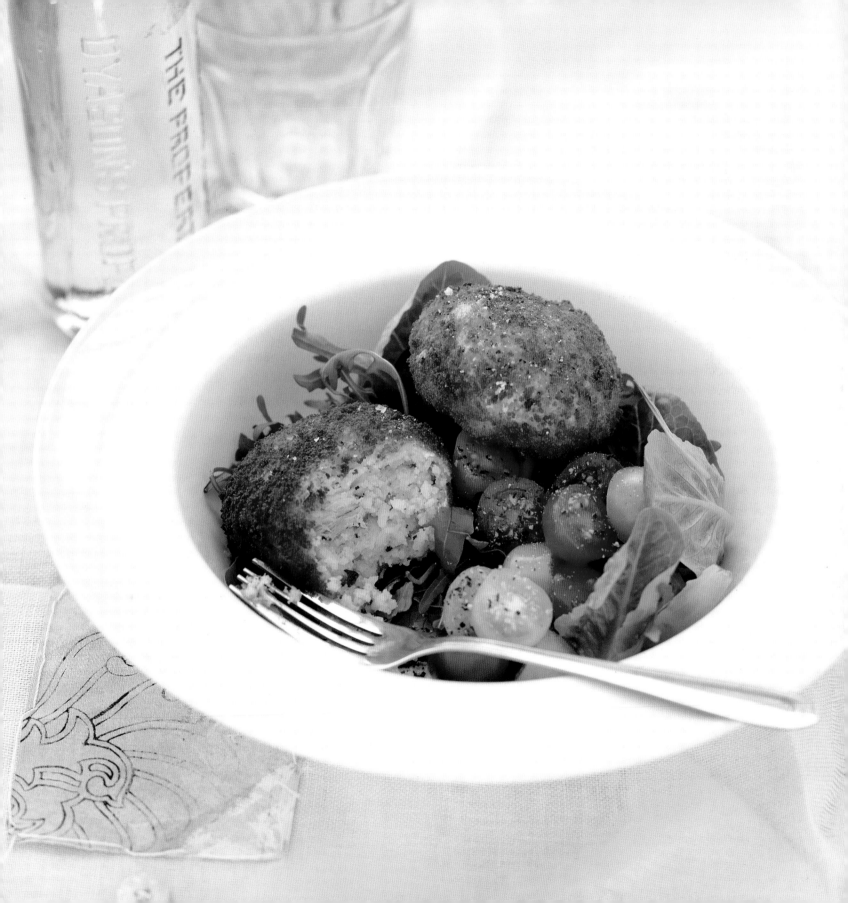

Lemon oregano chicken legs

SERVES 4

These delicious chicken legs are so easy to prepare and wonderfully versatile – enjoy them as a main meal, as finger food at a party, or packed into a picnic hamper.

Use a small knife to pierce the chicken evenly all over.

Combine the oregano, lemon zest and oil in a large bowl. Add the chicken, season and toss to coat. Cover and refrigerate for 3–4 hours, turning regularly.

Preheat the oven to 230°C. Line two baking trays with baking paper.

Place the chicken pieces on the trays and bake for 10–15 minutes or until golden brown and cooked through.

Meanwhile, to make the Greek salad, place the lettuce, tomatoes, olives and fetta in a large bowl and gently toss. Place the oil and vinegar in a small screw-top jar and shake well to combine. Pour over the salad and briefly toss through. Serve with the chicken legs, garnished with extra oregano.

16 skinless chicken legs
3 tablespoons finely chopped oregano, plus extra to garnish
1 tablespoon finely grated lemon zest
2 tablespoons extra virgin olive oil
salt and freshly ground black pepper

GREEK SALAD
2 cups (120 g) shredded iceberg lettuce
12 cherry tomatoes, cut in half
½ cup (75 g) pitted kalamata olives
100 g fetta, cut into 1 cm cubes
2 tablespoons olive oil
2 teaspoons balsamic vinegar

Lemon chicken and rice soup

SERVES 4

Made from just a handful of ingredients, this light, zesty soup is bursting with flavour and really satisfying. Enjoy it all year round.

Heat the oil in a large heavy-based saucepan over medium–high heat. Add the chicken pieces and cook, stirring regularly, until the chicken is browned all over. Add 2 litres water and bring to the boil. Reduce the heat to medium–low, add the lemon zest and juice (including the extra juice) and simmer, covered, for 20–30 minutes.

Add the rice to the pan and cook for 10 minutes. Add the celery and cook for a further 5 minutes or until the rice is tender. Stir in the parsley, season to taste and serve immediately.

1 tablespoon olive oil
1 kg chicken thigh fillets, visible fat removed, sliced
grated zest and juice of 2 lemons
½ cup (125 ml) lemon juice, extra
1 cup (200 g) white rice
3 stalks celery, finely sliced
1 tablespoon chopped flat-leaf parsley
salt and freshly ground black pepper

Lemon oregano chicken legs →

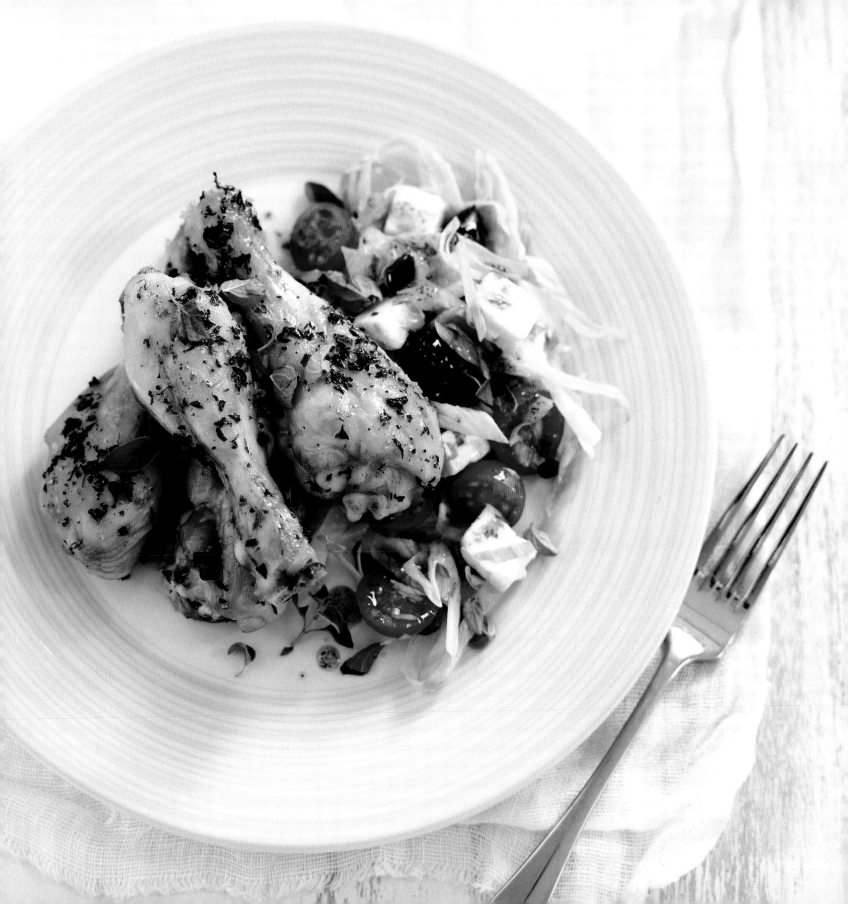

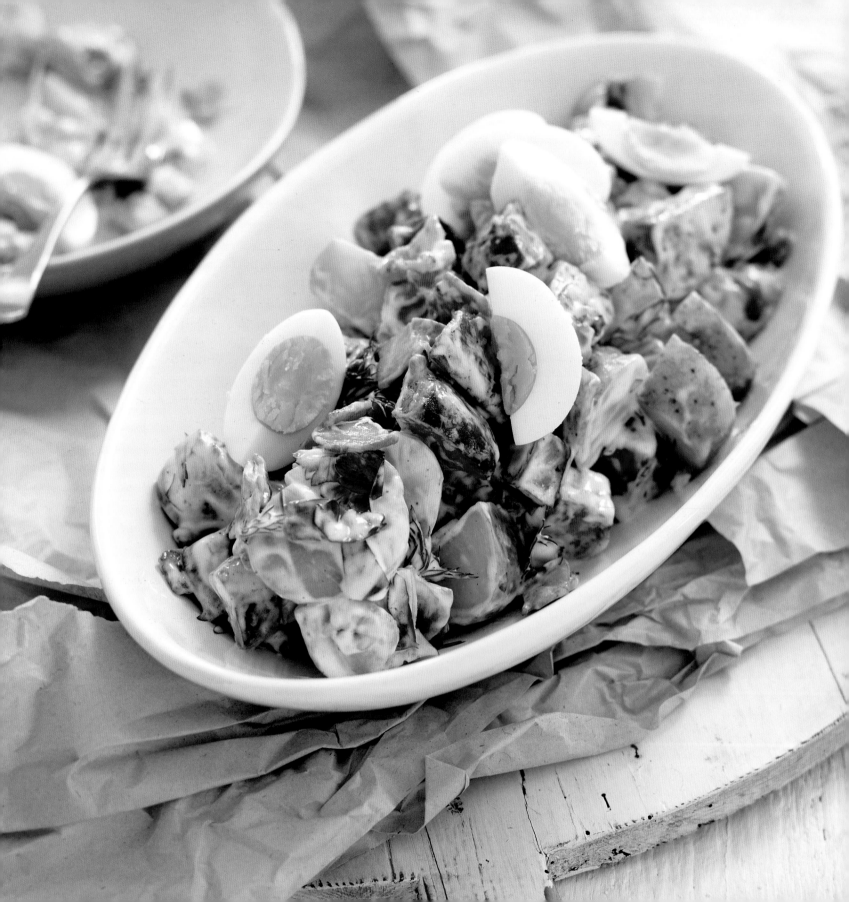

Mixed potato salad with bacon and herb dressing

SERVES 4–6

This is a nice twist on a traditional potato salad, with an added piquancy provided by the dill cucumbers and capers. It's sure to be a big hit at your next barbecue.

Preheat the oven to 180°C and line a baking tray with baking paper.

Place the sweet potato cubes on the baking tray, coat with a little canola oil and bake for 30 minutes, or until tender and golden. Remove from the oven, wrap in foil and cool to room temperature.

Meanwhile, place the potato in a large saucepan and cover with cold water. Bring to the boil and cook for 10–12 minutes or until the potato is tender when pierced with a skewer. Drain and cool to room temperature.

Cook the bacon in a small non-stick frying pan over high heat for about 3–4 minutes or until just crisp, stirring regularly. Remove from the heat.

In a small bowl, combine the mayonnaise, sour cream, dill cucumber, herbs, capers and bacon.

Place the cooled potato and sweet potato in a large bowl, then pour the mayonnaise mixture over the top and gently mix with a metal spoon. Season with salt and pepper. Gently stir to just combine, top with the egg and serve.

2 orange sweet potatoes, washed and cut into 2–3 cm cubes

1 tablespoon canola oil

6 potatoes, washed and cut into 2–3 cm cubes

6 rashers rindless bacon, trimmed of fat and chopped

125 g whole-egg mayonnaise (gluten-free if following a gluten-free diet)

100 g light sour cream

¾ cup (120 g) dill cucumbers, drained and finely chopped

1½ tablespoons chopped dill

3 tablespoons chopped flat-leaf parsley

1½ tablespoons capers

salt and freshly ground black pepper

2 eggs, hard-boiled and cut into quarters

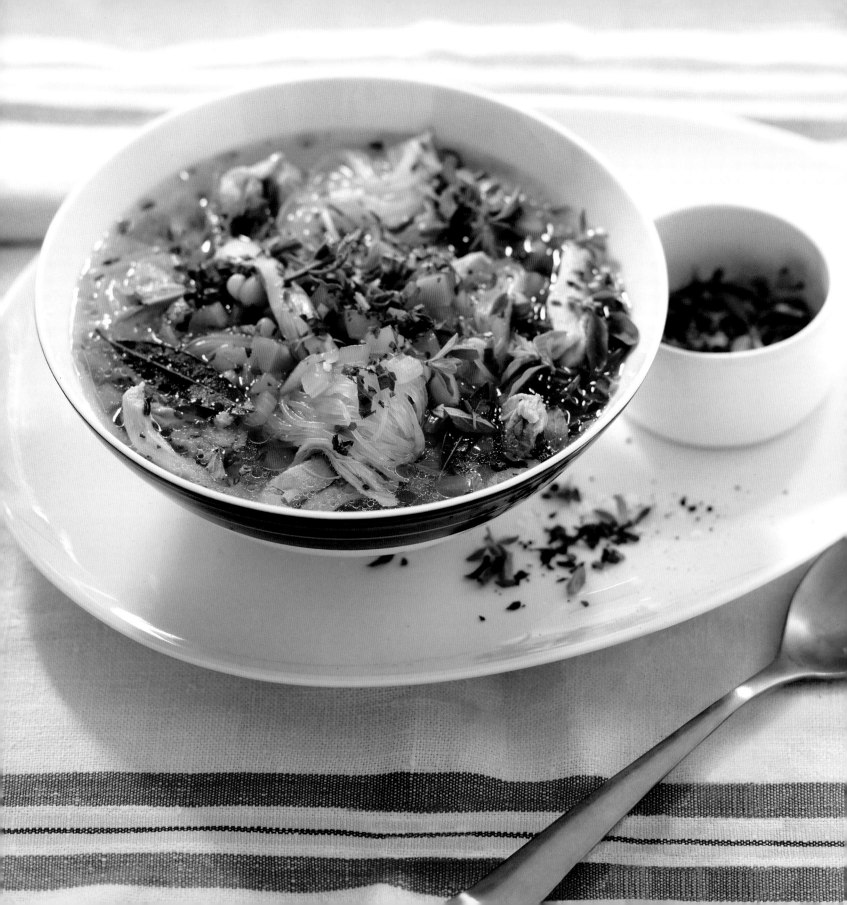

Chicken noodle and vegetable soup

SERVES 4

You can ask your butcher for chicken carcasses. They add a great natural flavour to the soup so you don't have to rely on stock cubes.

Heat the oil in a large saucepan over medium–high heat and cook the carrot, celery, bay leaf and turmeric for 10 minutes or until the vegetables have softened, stirring regularly.

Add the chicken carcasses, thyme and marjoram sprigs and 2.5 litres water. Bring to the boil, then reduce the heat and simmer, partially covered, for 1 hour. Remove the chicken carcasses and set aside for 10 minutes to cool. Strip the meat from the bones and shred into small pieces. Remove the bay leaf and herb sprigs. Bring the soup to a simmer over medium heat, then add the shredded chicken, sliced chicken thigh fillet and corn and cook for 8 minutes.

Meanwhile, soak the noodles in boiling water until soft. Drain.

Add the noodles to the soup and cook for a further 2 minutes. Stir in the thyme and marjoram, season to taste and serve with a sprinkling of parsley.

2 tablespoons canola oil
3 carrots, finely chopped
2 large stalks celery, finely chopped
1 bay leaf
½ teaspoon ground turmeric
1 kg chicken carcasses
5 sprigs of thyme
3 sprigs of marjoram
300 g chicken thigh fillets, thinly sliced
240 g tinned corn kernels, drained
1 cup (50 g) rice vermicelli noodles, broken into short lengths
1 tablespoon finely chopped thyme
2 teaspoons chopped marjoram
salt and freshly ground black pepper
2 tablespoons finely chopped flat-leaf parsley

Fetta, pumpkin and chive fritters

SERVES 4

Pumpkin and cumin work so well together, and the addition of salty fetta makes these fritters quite irresistible. Eat them just as they are or serve them with salad and a little sour cream for dipping.

Cook the pumpkin in a medium saucepan of boiling water for 8–10 minutes or until soft. Drain and mash, then set aside to cool.

Sift the flours and xanthan gum into a large mixing bowl. Add the chives, fetta, mashed pumpkin, egg and cumin and mix well with a metal spoon. Season with salt and pepper.

Heat 1 tablespoon oil in a medium non-stick frying pan over medium heat. Add 2 heaped tablespoons batter per fritter and cook for 2–3 minutes. Flip over and flatten slightly with the back of a spatula, then cook for a further 2 minutes or until golden brown and cooked through.

Remove the fritters to a plate and cover with foil to keep warm if eating immediately (otherwise store them in the fridge for later). Repeat with the remaining oil and batter until all the fritters are cooked.

Mix together the sour cream and extra chives. Serve the fritters with salad and a dollop of the sour cream mixture.

300 g pumpkin (squash), cut into 2 cm pieces
50 g fine rice flour
2 tablespoons maize cornflour
½ teaspoon xanthan gum
2 tablespoons chopped chives
60 g fetta, crumbled
2 eggs, lightly beaten
½–1 teaspoon ground cumin (to taste)
salt and freshly ground black pepper
2 tablespoons canola oil
3 tablespoons light sour cream
1 tablespoon chopped chives, extra
garden salad, to serve

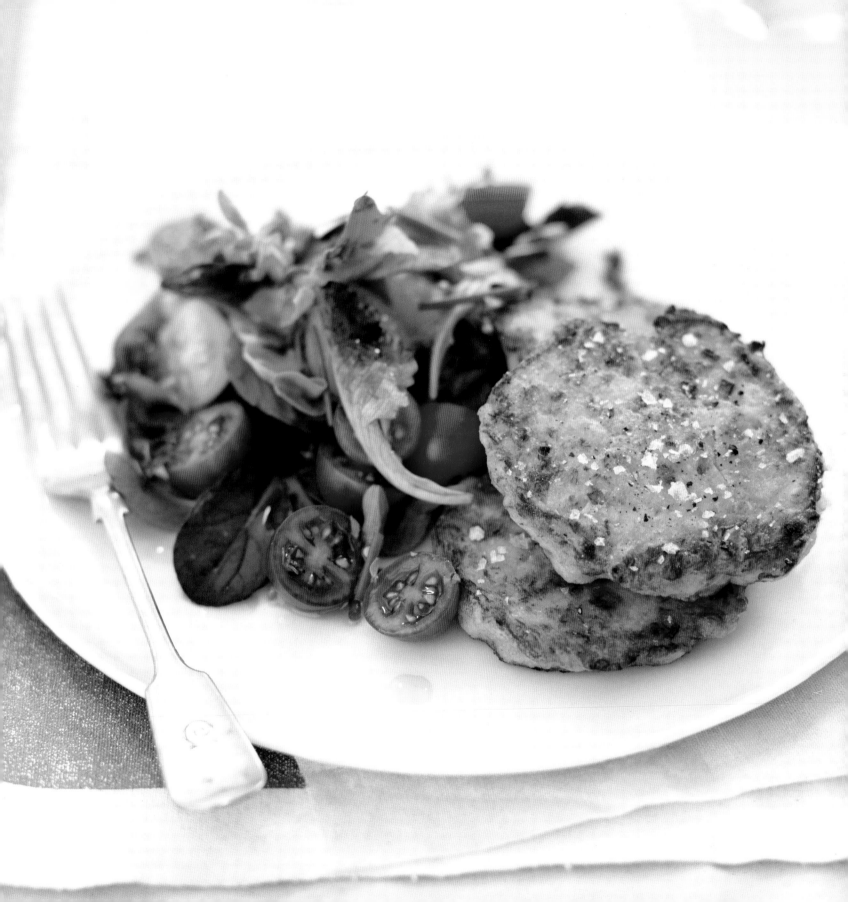

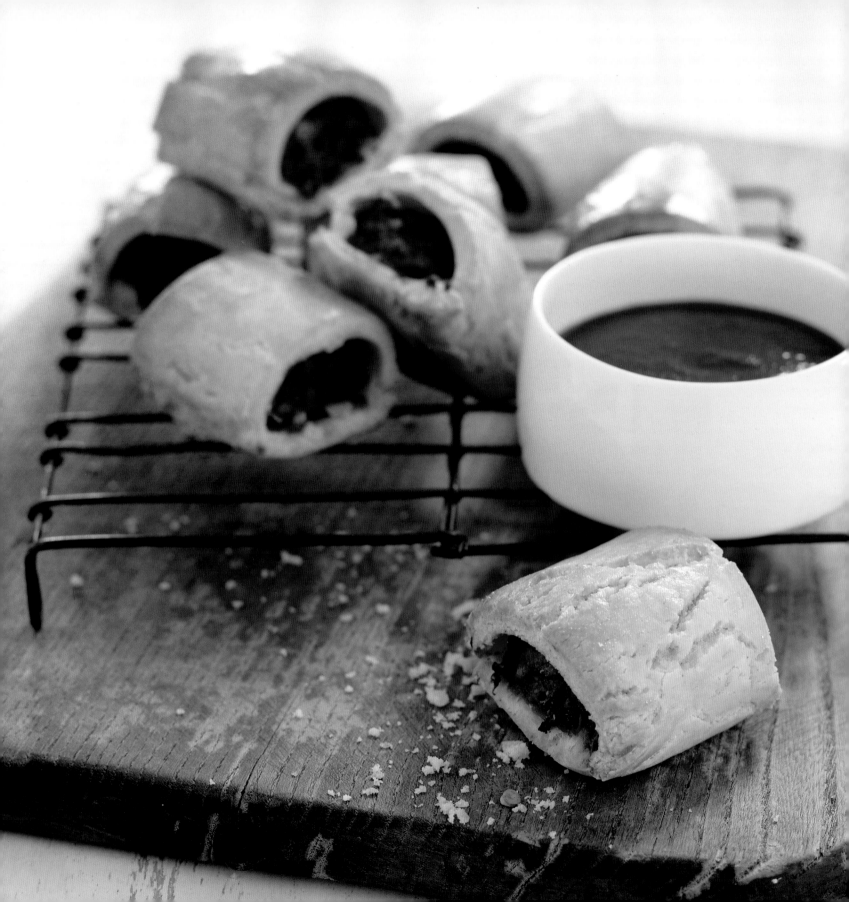

Sausage rolls

SERVES 4

Traditional sausage mince usually contains wheat fillers as a binder, and often contains onion. However, most larger supermarkets now stock suitable low-FODMAP sausage mince. The amount of soy flour used in this recipe is minimal so it will suit most people following the Low-FODMAP Diet. Assess your individual tolerance.

Preheat the oven to 170°C and lightly grease a baking tray.

To make the pastry, sift the flours and xanthan gum three times into a bowl (or mix well with a whisk to ensure they are well combined). Transfer to a food processor, add the butter and process until the mixture resembles fine breadcrumbs. While the motor is running, add the iced water (a tablespoon at a time) to form a soft dough. You may not need all the water. Turn out onto a bench dusted with gluten-free cornflour and knead until smooth. Wrap in plastic film and refrigerate for 30 minutes.

Place the dough between two sheets of baking paper and roll out to a rectangle about 20 cm long, with a thickness of 3–5 mm. Cut the rectangle in half lengthways.

In a small bowl, combine the mustard, oregano and 1 tablespoon warm water. Brush evenly over the rolled pastry.

Place half the sausage mince in a long line down the full length of each portion of pastry, about 1 cm from the edge. Roll the pastry to completely enclose the filling. Use a knife to trim the edges.

Cut the logs into 5 cm pieces. Brush with beaten egg and place on the prepared baking tray, then bake for 20–25 minutes or until cooked through and golden brown. Serve with tomato sauce, if liked.

1 teaspoon Dijon mustard (gluten-free if following a gluten-free diet)
½ teaspoon ground oregano
300 g gluten-free onion-free sausage mince
1 egg, lightly beaten
onion-free tomato sauce, to serve (optional)

PASTRY

1 cup (130 g) fine rice flour
½ cup (75 g) maize cornflour, plus extra for dusting
½ cup (45 g) debittered soy flour
1 teaspoon xanthan gum
160 g butter, chopped
60–100 ml iced water

Cream of potato and parsnip soup

SERVES 4

Many prepared stocks (cubes, powder and liquids) can contain onion. If this is a problem for you, make sure you read the labels carefully to ensure they are suitable.

Heat the oil in a medium saucepan over medium–low heat and cook the celery for 5–6 minutes until softened and golden brown. Add the parsnip and potato and cook, stirring, for 1–2 minutes. Pour in the stock and bring to the boil, then reduce the heat and simmer, covered, for 15–20 minutes or until the vegetables are tender. Remove from the heat and set aside for 10 minutes to cool a little.

Pour the vegetables and stock into a food processor. Add the milk and fetta and blend until smooth. Return to the cleaned saucepan and stir over medium heat until just below boiling point. Remove from the heat and season with salt and pepper. Ladle into four bowls and sprinkle with chopped chives.

1 tablespoon canola oil

1 stalk celery, very thinly sliced

6 parsnips, finely diced

2 potatoes, finely diced

3 cups (750 ml) onion-free vegetable stock (gluten-free if following a gluten-free diet)

½ cup (125 ml) low-fat milk

80 g fetta, crumbled

salt and freshly ground black pepper

2 tablespoons chopped chives

Chicken salad with herb dressing

SERVES 4

We all know that fresh herbs enhance the flavour of a dish, but they are also packed full of antioxidants. It's a win-win situation, so I try to add chopped herbs to my recipes as often as possible.

Heat 1 tablespoon oil in a large frying pan over medium heat and cook the chicken fillets for 4 minutes each side until golden brown and cooked through. Remove and cool to room temperature.

Place the mayonnaise, yoghurt, coriander, parsley and 1 tablespoon lemon juice in a small bowl and stir with a metal spoon until well combined.

Shred the cooled chicken into bite-sized pieces and mix through the mayonnaise dressing.

Place the lemon zest, remaining oil and remaining lemon juice in a small screw-top jar and shake well to combine.

Place the spinach leaves in a large bowl, add the lemon oil dressing and toss to coat. Divide the leaves among four bowls and top with the chicken mixture. Sprinkle with toasted almond flakes just before serving.

2 tablespoons extra virgin olive oil

4 × 150 g skinless chicken breast fillets

3 tablespoons whole-egg mayonnaise (gluten-free if following a gluten-free diet)

3 tablespoons natural yoghurt

1 tablespoon finely chopped coriander

2 tablespoons chopped flat-leaf parsley

3 tablespoons lemon juice

grated zest of 1 lemon

2 cups (40 g) baby spinach leaves

toasted almond flakes, to garnish

Gluten-free fatoush salad with chicken

SERVES 4

Gluten-free flatbreads are now readily available in the bread section of larger supermarkets, and may also be found in health-food stores. The main thing with this recipe is to add the toasted flatbread just before serving, otherwise it will go soggy.

Mix together the cumin and 1 tablespoon vegetable oil in a small bowl and brush over all sides of the chicken fillets. Wrap in plastic film and marinate in the fridge for about 30 minutes.

Preheat the oven to 160°C. Place the flatbreads on a baking tray and bake for 5 minutes or until just crisp and lightly golden. Break into bite-sized pieces and set aside.

Place the cucumber, tomato, capsicum and chopped herbs in a large bowl and toss to combine.

To make the dressing, place all the ingredients in a small screw-top jar and shake well to combine.

Heat the remaining vegetable oil in a medium frying pan over medium heat. Add the chicken fillets and cook for 3–4 minutes each side or until just cooked through. Remove and rest for 5 minutes, then cut into rough cubes.

Add the crisp flatbread, chicken and dressing to the salad, toss gently and serve immediately.

1 tablespoon ground cumin

1½ tablespoons vegetable oil

2 × 160 g skinless chicken breast fillets

3 × 20 cm round gluten-free flatbreads

2 small cucumbers, cut in half lengthways, sliced

2 tomatoes, chopped

½ red capsicum (pepper), chopped

½ green capsicum (pepper), chopped

½ cup (15 g) chopped flat-leaf parsley

3 tablespoons chopped mint

SPICED LEMON DRESSING

3 tablespoons olive oil

2 tablespoons lemon juice

1 tablespoon garlic-infused canola oil

1 teaspoon ground cinnamon

1 tablespoon ground cumin

1 teaspoon ground coriander

salt and freshly ground black pepper

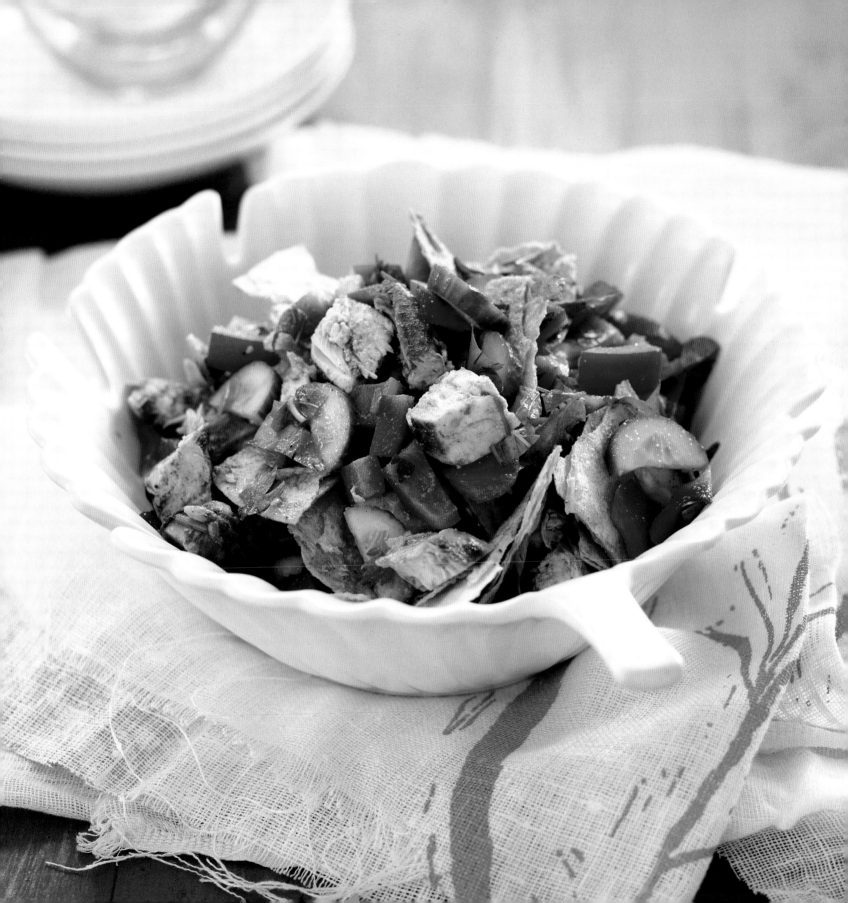

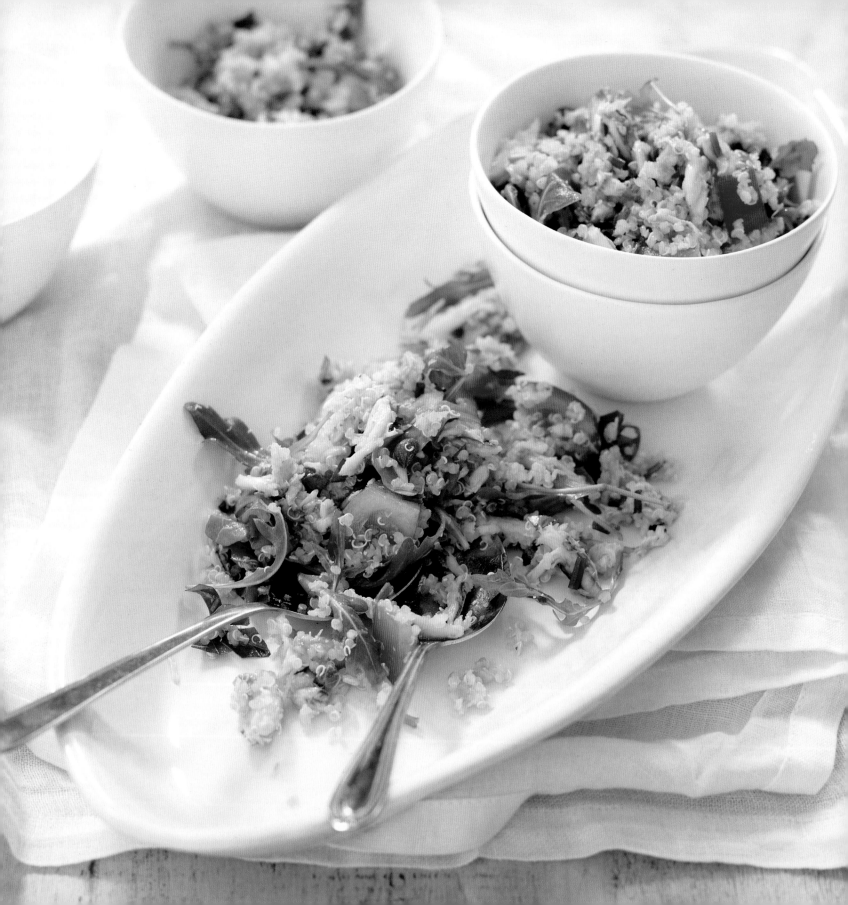

Crab and rocket quinoa salad

SERVES 4

This recipe uses quinoa, an ancient gluten-free grain that is full of nutrients. It has a texture similar to cracked wheat (bulgur) – in fact, in many recipes the two are interchangeable.

Pour 2 cups (500 ml) water into a small saucepan and bring to the boil over medium–high heat. Reduce the heat to medium and add the quinoa. Cook, stirring regularly, for 10–15 minutes or until all the water has been absorbed and the quinoa is tender. Set aside to cool to room temperature.

To make the herb dressing, place all the ingredients in a small screw-top jar and shake well to combine.

Combine the quinoa, tomato, crabmeat, rocket and dressing in a large bowl. Cover and refrigerate for 20–30 minutes to allow the flavours to infuse.

½ cup (50 g) dried quinoa
2 tomatoes, chopped
300 g tinned crabmeat
2 cups (40 g) rocket leaves

HERB DRESSING
3 tablespoons extra virgin olive oil
1 tablespoon lemon juice
1 teaspoon grated lemon zest
½ teaspoon finely chopped red chilli
1 tablespoon capers, drained
2 tablespoons roughly chopped
  flat-leaf parsley
2 tablespoons chopped chives

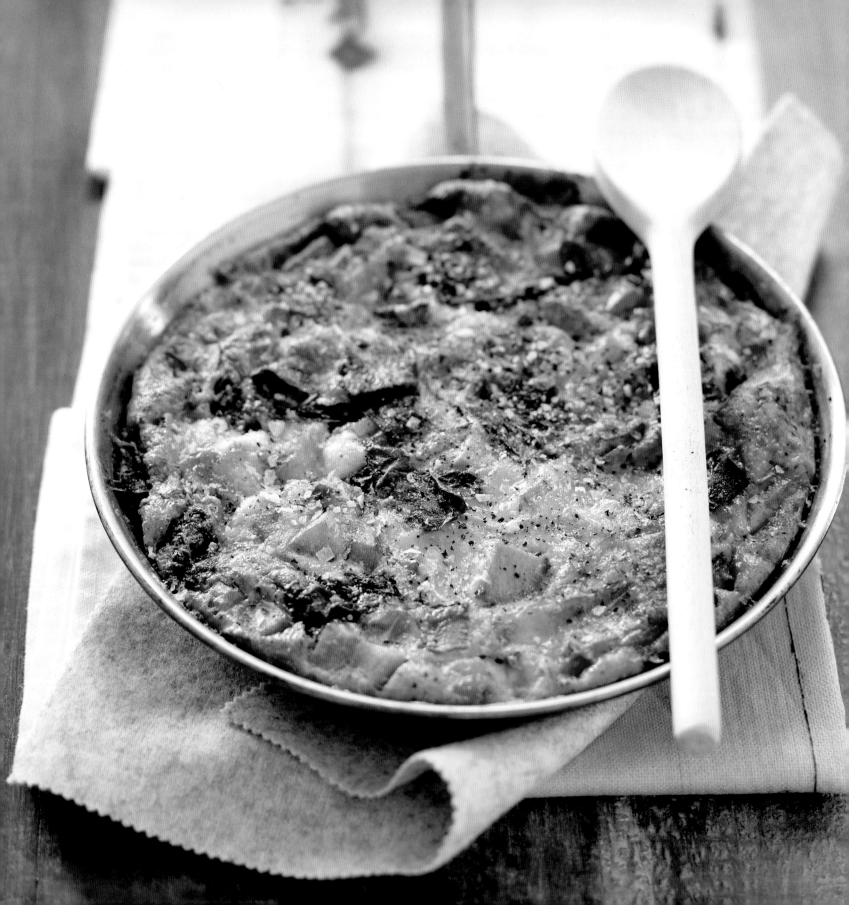

Sweet potato, blue cheese and spinach frittata

SERVES 4

Frittatas are so versatile. You can add whatever ingredients you like to the egg base (although the combination below is just delicious), then serve them hot, cold or at room temperature for lunch or dinner, or as finger food. If you don't have an ovenproof frying pan, fry the sweet potato then transfer it to a greased 18 cm baking dish. Pour the egg mixture over the top and proceed with the recipe.

20 g butter
2 sweet potatoes, cut into 1 cm cubes
2 cups (40 g) baby spinach leaves
100 g strong blue cheese
8 eggs, lightly beaten
salt and freshly ground black pepper
salad, to serve

Preheat the oven to 180°C.

Melt the butter in an 18 cm frying pan with an ovenproof handle over medium heat. Add the sweet potato cubes and cook for 10 minutes or until tender and golden brown.

Lightly whisk together the spinach, blue cheese and egg in a bowl. Pour over the sweet potato, then place the pan in the oven and bake for 20–25 minutes or until firm (test by gently wobbling the pan).

Remove from the oven, then leave for 5 minutes before slicing. Serve with salad.

Pork and crunchy noodle salad

SERVES 4

More often than not, noodles are made from wheat. However, gluten-free fried noodles are now available in the packet noodle section of most major supermarkets. Here, they add a great texture to the salad.

Mix together the oil, five-spice powder, fish sauce, vinegar, ginger and brown sugar in a non-metallic bowl. Add the pork strips and toss until well coated in the marinade. Cover and refrigerate for about 3 hours.

Heat the sesame oil in a wok over medium heat. Add the pork and any leftover marinade and cook until just cooked through – don't overcook or the meat will not be tender.

In a large bowl, combine the remaining ingredients with the pork strips and cooking juices. Divide among four bowls and serve immediately.

1 tablespoon garlic-infused canola oil

3 teaspoons Chinese five-spice powder

3 tablespoons fish sauce

3 tablespoons sushi vinegar

2 teaspoons grated ginger

3 teaspoons brown sugar

400 g pork butterfly steak,
    cut into thin strips

2 tablespoons sesame oil

5 cups (150 g) roughly chopped
    iceberg lettuce

1 cup (50 g) snowpea sprouts

½ large cucumber, diced

2 stalks celery, thinly sliced

½ green capsicum (pepper), diced

½ cup (25 g) chopped coriander
    or Vietnamese mint

100 g fried rice noodles

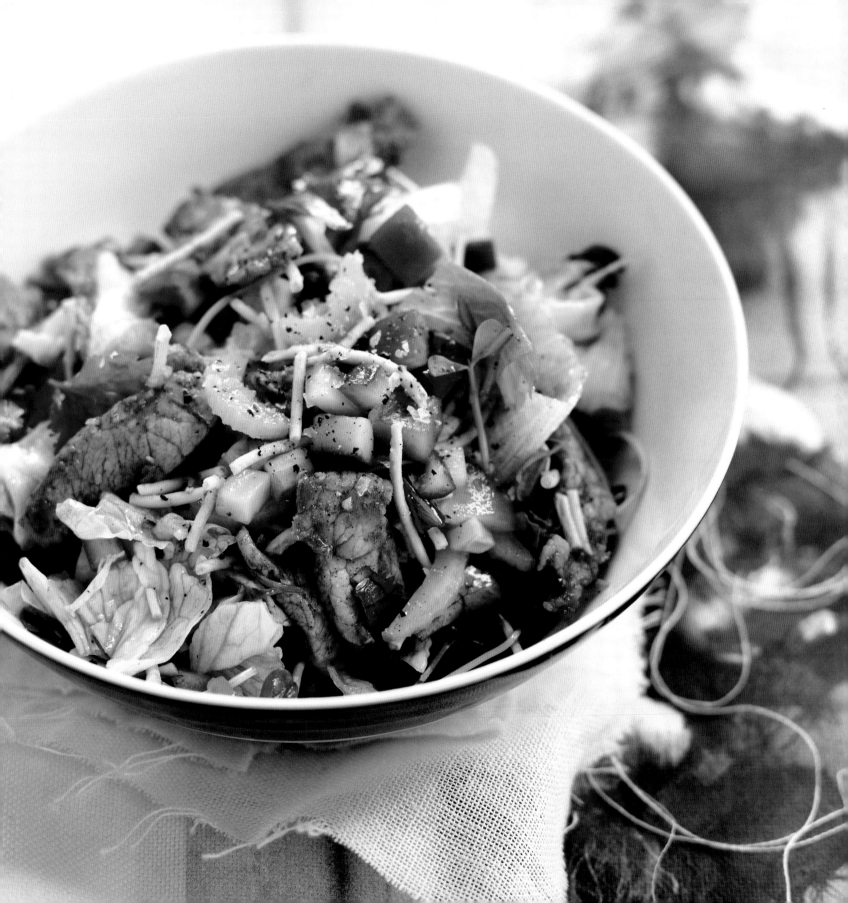

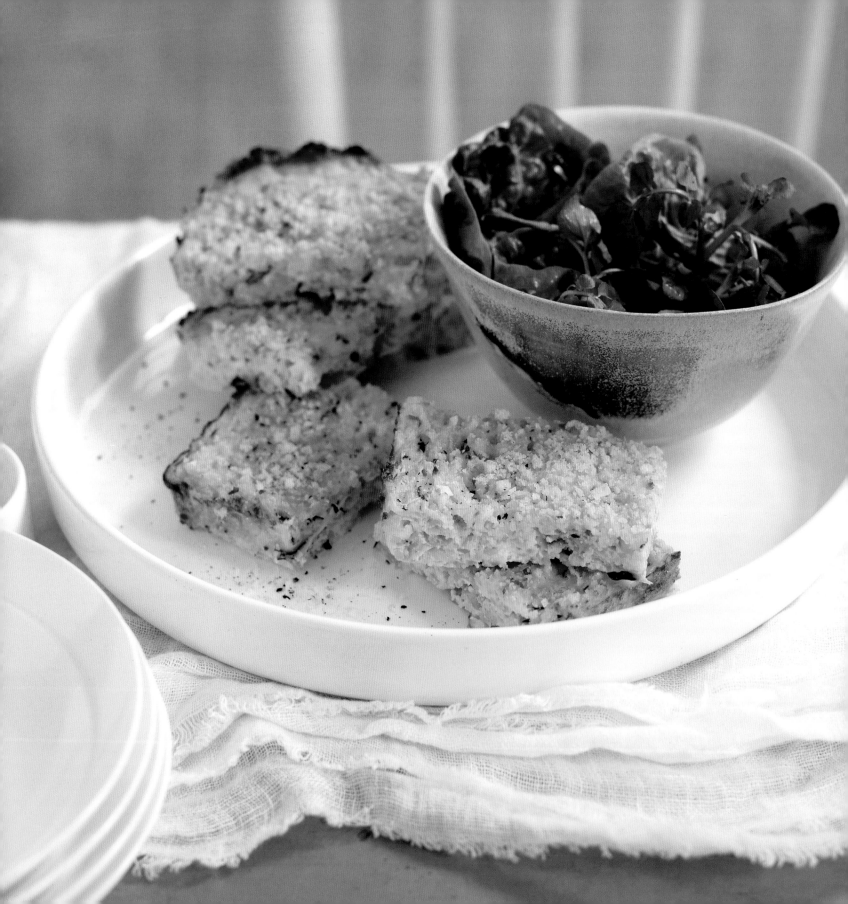

Pumpkin, rice and ricotta slice

SERVES 6–8

This delicious rice-based dish cooks up to make a firm slice, which may be enjoyed as a light meal or cut into bite-sized pieces to serve as finger food. For those with lactose intolerance, replace the ricotta with fetta.

Preheat the oven to 180°C. Grease a 22 cm square ovenproof dish and sprinkle half the breadcrumbs around the base and sides. Invert the dish and shake away any excess crumbs.

Bring 2 cups (500 ml) water to the boil in a medium saucepan, add the rice and cook over medium–high heat for 12–15 minutes or until tender. Drain, then return the rice to the pan and stir in the grated pumpkin and zucchini. Cover and set aside.

Combine the egg and cheeses in a small bowl and season with salt and pepper. Add the rice mixture and stir until well combined. Spoon into the prepared dish and sprinkle the remaining breadcrumbs over the top. Bake for 45–55 minutes or until firm on top when pressed. Remove from the oven and set aside for 5–10 minutes before cutting into pieces. Serve with salad.

35 g fresh gluten-free breadcrumbs (made from day-old bread)
⅓ cup (65 g) arborio rice
200 g grated pumpkin (squash)
1 zucchini (courgette), grated
2 eggs, lightly beaten
200 g firm fresh ricotta
⅔ cup (50 g) grated parmesan
salt and freshly ground black pepper
green salad, to serve

Goat's cheese and chive souffles

MAKES 6

Baking a souffle might seem like a daunting task, but it needn't be.
I guarantee this dairy-free dish will be a great success – try it for your
next dinner party! For those with lactose intolerance, replace the goat's
milk with lactose-free milk.

Preheat the oven to 180°C and line a baking tray with baking paper. Grease six
150 ml souffle dishes and lightly coat with gluten-free breadcrumbs. Invert the
dishes and shake away any excess crumbs.

Melt the margarine in a medium saucepan over low heat. Add the cornflour
and cook, stirring constantly, for 1–2 minutes. Slowly pour in the goat's milk
and mix to make a smooth paste. Cook, stirring, for a further 2–3 minutes or
until thickened.

Transfer the mixture to a medium bowl. Add the egg yolks, one at a time,
beating well with electric beaters between additions. Add the goat's cheese,
chives and parsley and beat until just combined. Season with salt and pepper.

In a large clean bowl, beat the egg whites with clean electric beaters until firm
peaks form. Gently fold into the cheese and herb mixture until well combined.
Spoon into the souffle dishes, then place the dishes in a shallow baking dish.
Pour enough boiling water into the baking dish to come halfway up the sides
of the dishes. Bake for 20 minutes or until well risen and slightly browned.

To make the topping, combine the breadcrumbs, chives and goat's cheese
in a small bowl. Season with salt and mix to a fine texture.

Remove the souffles from the oven and place them on the prepared tray.
Brush with melted margarine and sprinkle with the breadcrumb topping. Bake
for a further 7–8 minutes or until puffed with a firm crust. Serve immediately
with salad, if liked.

3 tablespoons dried gluten-free
breadcrumbs
60 g dairy-free margarine, plus extra
for brushing
⅓ cup (50 g) maize cornflour
300 ml goat's milk
3 large eggs, separated
120 g goat's cheese, crumbled
2 teaspoons chopped chives
2 teaspoons finely chopped
flat-leaf parsley
salt and freshly ground black pepper
green salad, to serve (optional)

TOPPING

2 tablespoons fresh gluten-free
breadcrumbs (made from
day-old bread)
1 teaspoon chopped chives
20 g goat's cheese
salt

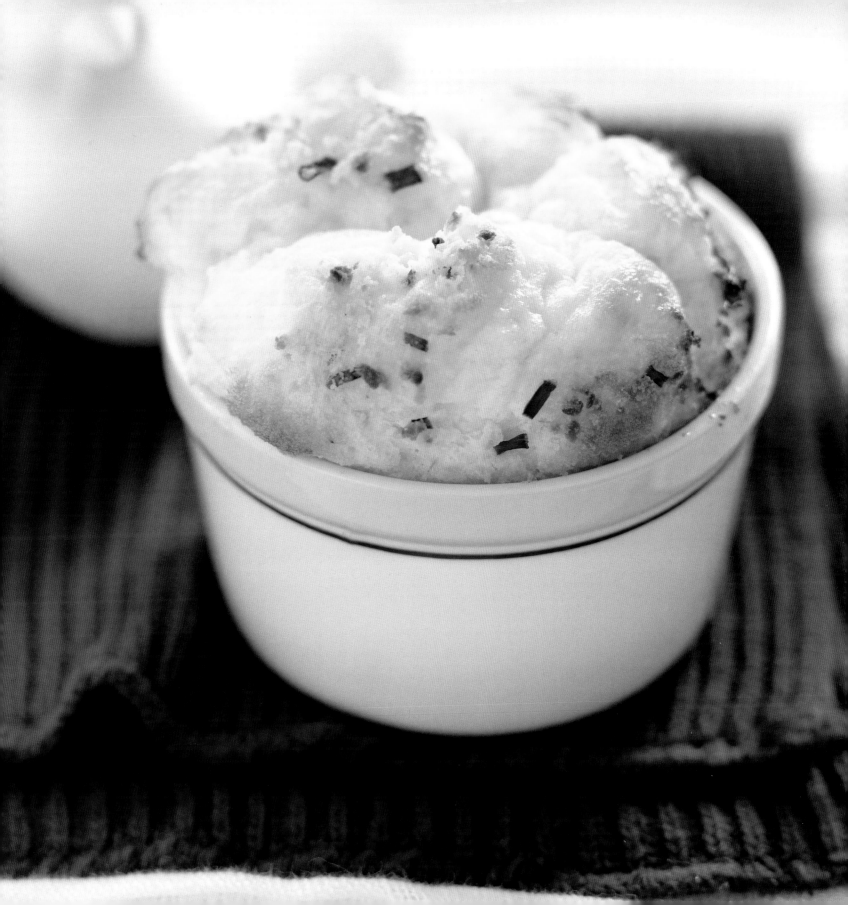

Zucchini and potato torte

SERVES 6

This delicious dish can be served hot or cold. Children love it too,
so it is a great one to pack into school lunchboxes.

Preheat the oven to 170°C. Lightly grease an 18 cm square baking dish.

Cook the potatoes in a saucepan of lightly salted water for 10–15 minutes
or until tender. Drain. When cool enough to handle, cut into 3 mm thick slices.
Layer the potato slices over the base of the baking dish.

Combine the remaining ingredients in a large bowl and pour over the potato
slices, shaking the dish to ensure the mixture is evenly distributed through the
potato. Bake for 45–50 minutes or until golden and cooked through. Remove
from the oven and leave for 5–10 minutes before slicing and serving.

3 potatoes, peeled
2 large zucchini (courgettes), grated
200 g bacon or prosciutto, diced
1½ cups (180 g) grated low-fat cheddar
½ cup (75 g) maize cornflour
2 tablespoons canola oil
6 eggs, lightly beaten
salt and freshly ground black pepper

Egg and spinach salad

SERVES 4

This simple salad is a superb alternative to a green garden salad. The egg gives flavour and colour, and the sesame dressing adds a wonderful toastiness.

Heat 2 teaspoons sesame oil in a medium non-stick frying pan over medium–high heat and add half the beaten egg. Tilt the pan to form a thin pancake and cook for about 1 minute until just cooked through. Remove from the pan and repeat with the remaining oil and beaten egg. Allow the pancakes to cool, then slice into large diamond strips.

   To make the dressing, combine all the ingredients in a small bowl.

   Place the spinach, snowpea sprouts, capsicum and egg strips in a large bowl and toss gently to combine. Divide among four serving bowls, drizzle the dressing over the top and serve.

1 tablespoon sesame oil

4 eggs, beaten

300 g baby spinach leaves

100 g snowpea sprouts

1 green capsicum (pepper), sliced into 2 cm lengths

DRESSING

1½ tablespoons soy sauce (gluten-free if following a gluten-free diet)

2 tablespoons lemon juice

2 tablespoons sesame oil

1½ tablespoons brown sugar

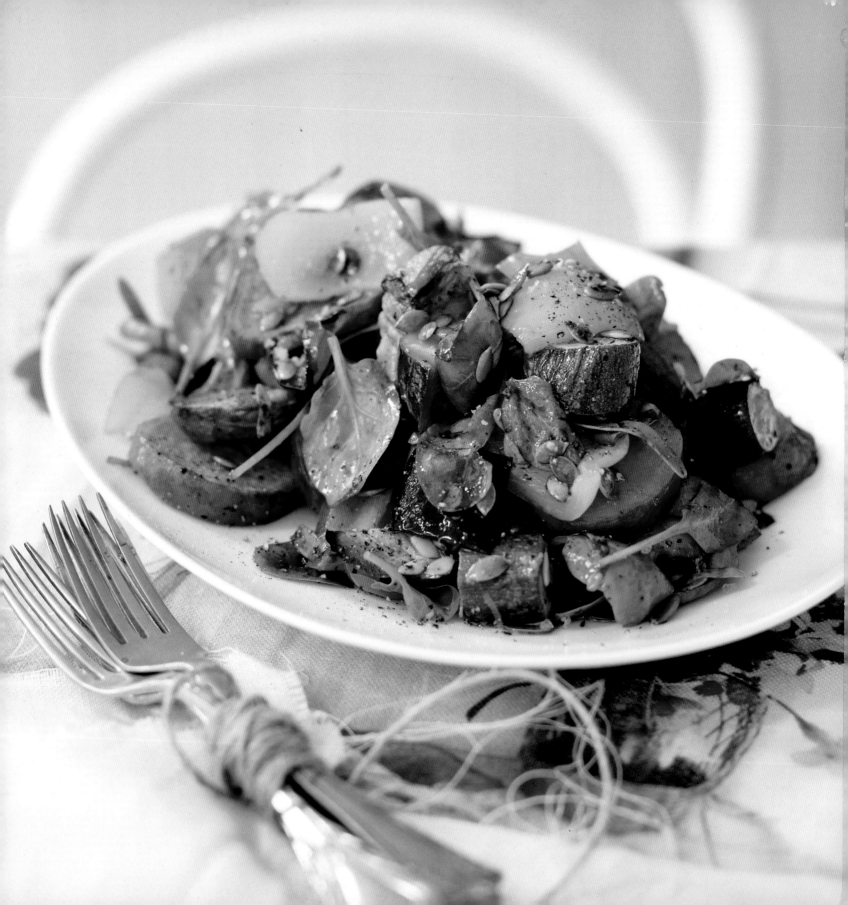

Roast vegetable salad

SERVES 4

This colourful array of roast vegetables is rich in antioxidants, has a delicious caramelised flavour and looks great on the plate. With this winning combination, it is sure to become one of your favourite salads.

Preheat the oven to 200°C and line two baking trays with baking paper.

Combine the vegetables in a large bowl, pour over a little oil and toss to coat. Place the vegetable pieces on the trays in a single layer and roast for 20 minutes or until golden, turning occasionally to ensure even browning. Remove from the oven. Cover with foil and cool to room temperature, then place in the refrigerator for 30 minutes.

To make the dressing, place all the ingredients in a small screw-top jar and shake well to combine.

Combine the cooled vegetables and spinach in a large bowl. Add the dressing and toss well, then season to taste with salt and pepper.

1 eggplant (aubergine), cut into
 4 cm cubes
2 zucchini (courgettes), cut into
 thick slices
1 red capsicum (pepper), cut into
 4 cm cubes
1 yellow capsicum (pepper),
 cut into 4 cm cubes
2 large sweet potatoes, cut into
 1 cm thick rounds
300 g pumpkin (squash), cut into
 2 cm cubes
garlic-infused olive oil, for coating
3 cups (60 g) baby spinach leaves
salt and freshly ground black pepper

BALSAMIC DRESSING

2 teaspoons balsamic vinegar
3 tablespoons garlic-infused olive oil
2 tablespoons pepitas

Chicken tikka skewers

SERVES 6

If you are using wooden skewers, it is important to soak them in water before adding the chicken – this will prevent them from scorching under the grill. These delicious skewers may also be threaded onto sturdy toothpicks and served as finger food.

Combine the yoghurt, ginger, garam masala, cumin, coriander, turmeric and chilli in a large bowl and season with salt and pepper. Add the chicken pieces and stir to ensure they are evenly coated. Cover with plastic film and refrigerate for 2 hours.

Thread the chicken pieces onto 18 skewers. Place under a hot grill, turning to cook all sides until golden brown and just cooked through. Serve with salad.

200 g Greek-style yoghurt
1 tablespoon finely grated ginger
3 teaspoons garam masala
¼ teaspoon ground cumin
¼ teaspoon ground coriander
2 teaspoons ground turmeric
¼–½ teaspoon ground chilli
salt and freshly ground black pepper
1.2 kg chicken breast fillets, cut into
   2 cm cubes
green salad, to serve

Spiced tofu bites

SERVES 4

Tofu is a great vegetarian protein food and is tolerated by most people on the Low-FODMAP Diet. Assess your individual tolerance. This dish uses light, airy tofu puffs, which are available vacuum-packed in the refrigerator section of Asian grocers.

Combine the caraway seeds, pepper, salt, paprika and allspice in a small bowl and stir in 2 tablespoons oil. Brush the spice mix over the tofu, then transfer to a plate. Cover and refrigerate for 2–3 hours to allow the flavours to infuse.

Heat the remaining oil in a medium frying pan over medium–high heat. Add the tofu and cook for 1–2 minutes each side or until warmed through. Serve with steamed rice and salad.

1 teaspoon ground caraway seeds
½ teaspoon freshly ground
   black pepper
½ teaspoon salt
¼ teaspoon paprika
¼ teaspoon ground allspice
⅓ cup (80 ml) vegetable oil
400 g puffed tofu pieces
   (about 5 cm × 5 cm)
steamed rice and salad, to serve

Chicken tikka skewers →

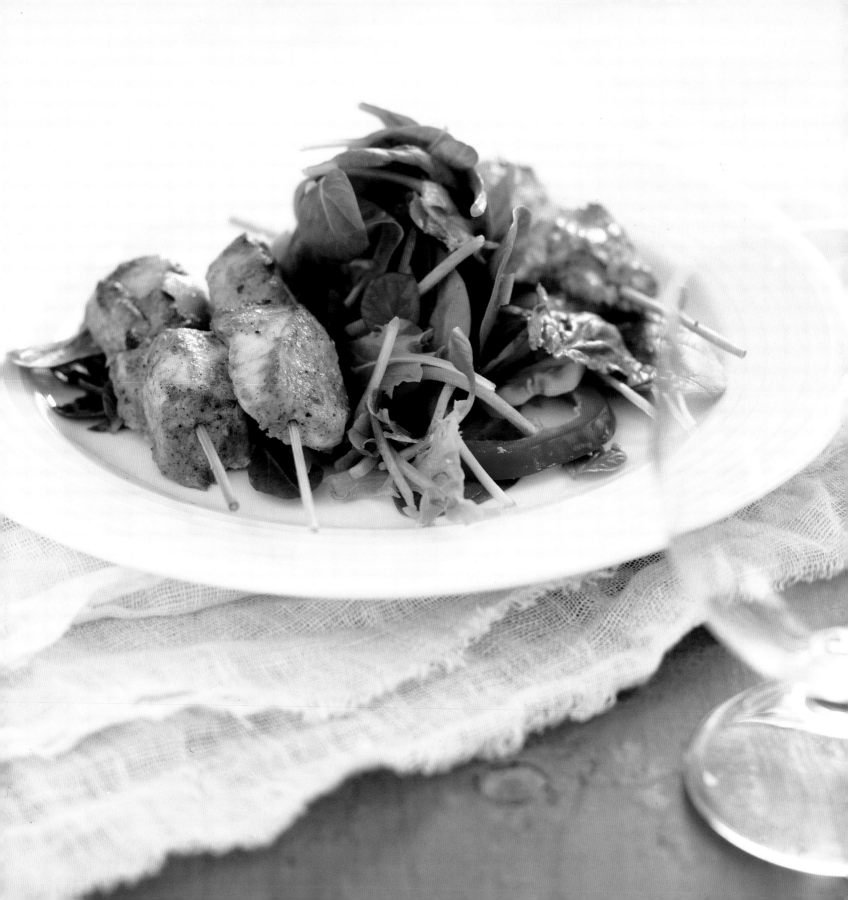

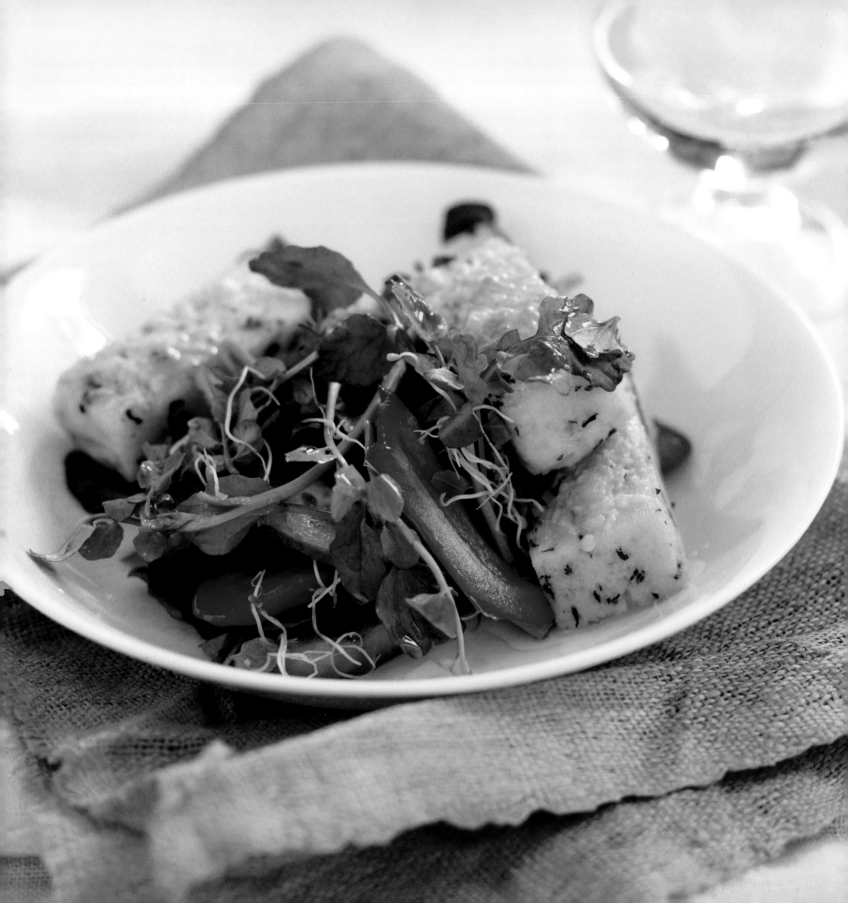

Cheese and herb polenta wedges with watercress salad

SERVES 4

Polenta is versatile, inexpensive and satisfying, yet many people have not experienced the pleasure of cooking with it. Here, the polenta is baked until firm, then cut into generous wedges (you could also cut it into smaller pieces to serve as nibbles). Enjoy it hot, cold or at room temperature.

Bring the stock to the boil in a medium saucepan. Pour in the polenta and cook over medium heat for 3–5 minutes, stirring constantly – the mixture should be very thick. Stir in the butter, herbs and half the parmesan.

Line a 15 cm square baking dish with baking paper. Pour the polenta into the dish and smooth the surface. Cool slightly and then refrigerate for 1 hour.

Preheat the oven to 180°C and line a baking tray with baking paper.

Turn out the polenta onto a chopping board and cut into eight wedges or rectangles. Place the wedges on the tray and sprinkle with the remaining parmesan. Bake for 10–15 minutes or until the cheese has melted and the wedges are lightly golden. Alternatively, cook under a hot grill for 5–7 minutes.

Meanwhile, to make the watercress salad, combine the watercress, cucumber, green and red capsicum and alfalfa in a large bowl. Drizzle with the lemon-infused oil and toss to combine. Serve with the warm polenta wedges.

3 cups (750 ml) onion-free vegetable stock (gluten-free if following a gluten-free diet)
1 cup (170 g) instant polenta
30 g butter
⅓ cup (10 g) chopped flat-leaf parsley
⅓ cup (10 g) chopped oregano
⅓ cup (10 g) chopped marjoram
½ cup (40 g) grated parmesan

WATERCRESS SALAD

4 cups (80 g) watercress
½ small cucumber, thinly sliced
½ green capsicum (pepper), cut into 2 cm strips
½ red capsicum (pepper), cut into 2 cm strips
3 tablespoons alfalfa sprouts
3 tablespoons lemon-infused olive oil

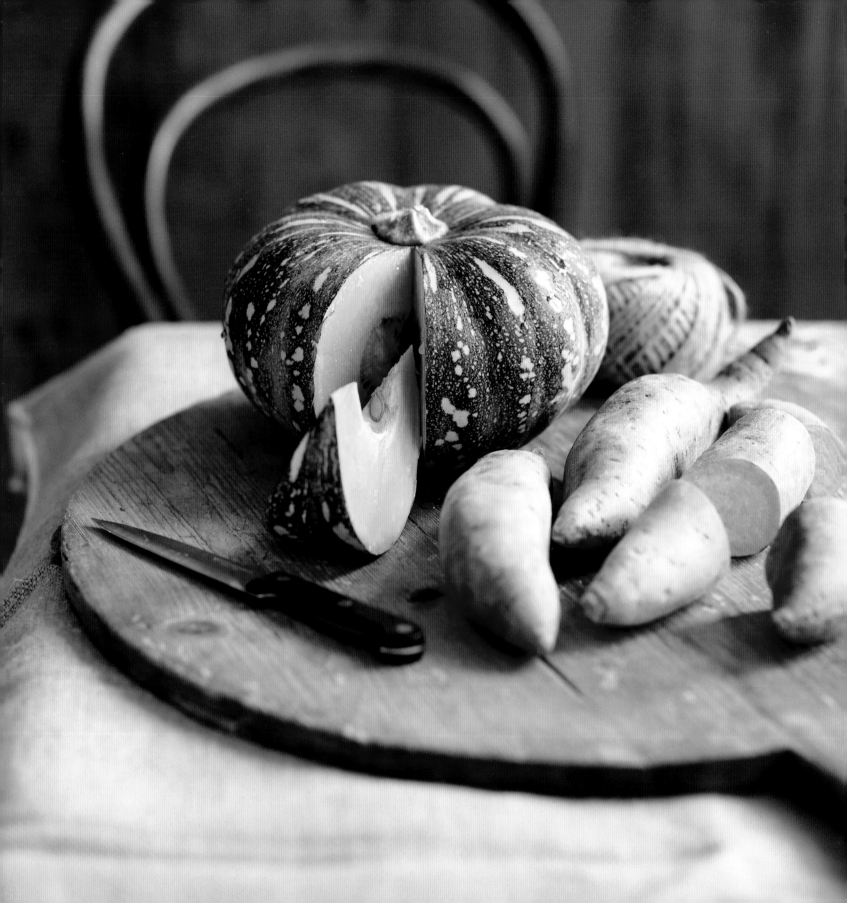

Main meals

Prosciutto chicken with sage polenta

SERVES 4

The creamy polenta is enhanced by the distinctive flavour of sage, providing a delicious flavour base for the chicken. If you are unable to purchase prosciutto, bacon will work just as well.

Preheat the oven to 180°C and line a baking tray with baking paper.

Wrap each chicken breast in a slice of prosciutto and secure with a toothpick. Place on the tray and bake for 20 minutes or until the chicken is cooked through and the prosciutto is crisp.

Meanwhile, to make the sage polenta, heat the milk and oil in a medium saucepan until almost boiling. Add the polenta and stir until the mixture boils. Reduce the heat to low and cook, stirring constantly, for a further 3–5 minutes until the polenta is cooked (it should be the texture of smooth mashed potato). Stir in the sage and season with salt and pepper.

Spoon the polenta onto four warmed serving plates and top with the prosciutto chicken. Sprinkle with extra sage leaves and serve.

4 × 200 g skinless chicken breast fillets
4 slices prosciutto

SAGE POLENTA
3 cups (750 ml) low-fat milk
2 tablespoons garlic-infused olive oil
⅔ cup (110 g) instant polenta
2 tablespoons sage leaves, torn if large, plus extra to serve
salt and freshly ground black pepper

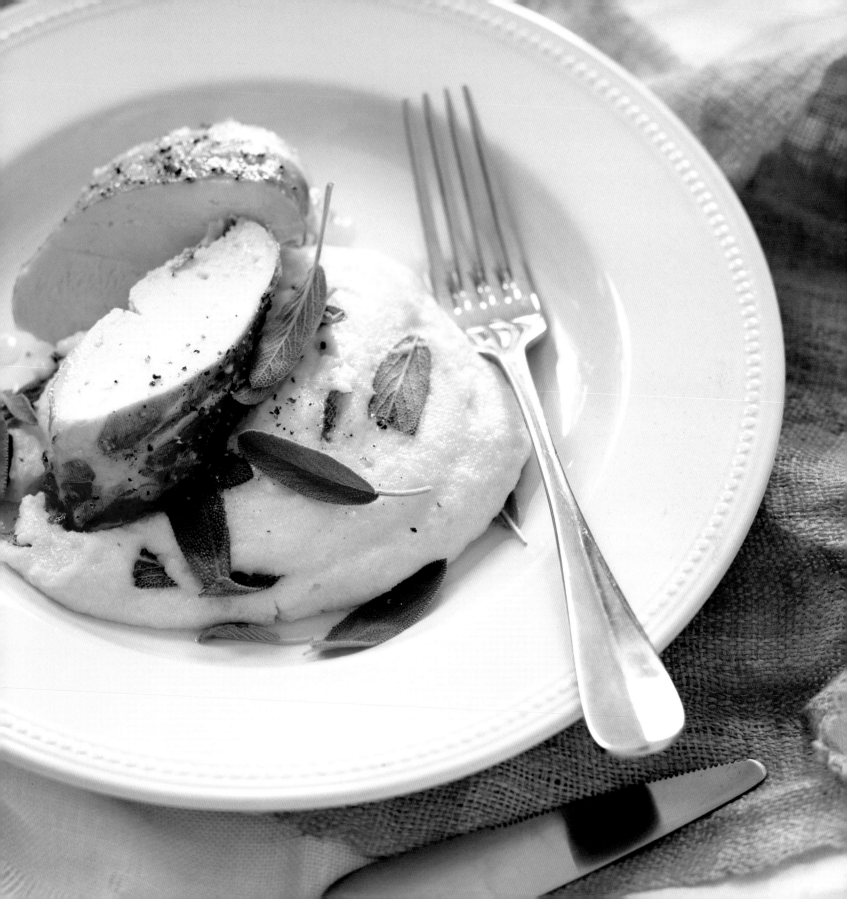

Fetta, spinach and pine nut crepes

SERVES 6

Soy flour is quite bitter in its uncooked state but the bitterness disappears when cooked. I prefer to use a debittered soy flour, although sometimes it can be a little difficult to track down. The amount of soy flour used in this recipe is minimal so it will suit most people following the Low-FODMAP Diet. Assess your individual tolerance – if necessary, you can replace the soy flour with tapioca flour.

Sift the flours and bicarbonate of soda three times into a bowl (or mix well with a whisk to ensure they are well combined) and make a well in the centre. Add the milk and beaten egg and blend to form a smooth batter. Stir in the melted butter. Cover with plastic film and set aside for 20 minutes.

Heat a heavy-based frying pan over medium heat and spray with cooking spray. Pour in enough batter to coat the base when the pan is tilted, and cook until bubbles appear. Turn and cook the other side, then remove and keep warm. Repeat with the remaining batter to make 12 crepes in all.

Preheat the oven to 180°C.

To make the filling, heat the oil in a large heavy-based frying pan over medium–high heat and cook the pine nuts until just browned (watch carefully as they can burn easily). Add the spinach and fetta and stir until well combined, then stir in the egg until just cooked. Season to taste.

Place spoonfuls of filling across the centre of each crepe and roll up. Place the rolled crepes, seam-side down, in one large or two small baking dishes in a single layer and pour the pureed tomato evenly over the top. Scatter with grated cheese and bake for 10–15 minutes or until the cheese has melted. Serve with salad, if liked.

¾ cup (100 g) fine rice flour

½ cup (75 g) maize cornflour

⅓ cup (30 g) debittered soy flour

¾ teaspoon bicarbonate of soda

1½ cups (375 ml) low-fat milk

2 eggs, lightly beaten

40 g butter, melted

cooking spray

1 cup (280 g) pureed tomato

½ cup (60 g) grated low-fat cheddar

salad, to serve (optional)

**FETTA, SPINACH AND
PINE NUT FILLING**

2 teaspoons canola oil

3 tablespoon pine nuts

500 g chopped frozen spinach, thawed

500 g fetta, crumbled

1 egg, lightly beaten

salt and freshly ground black pepper

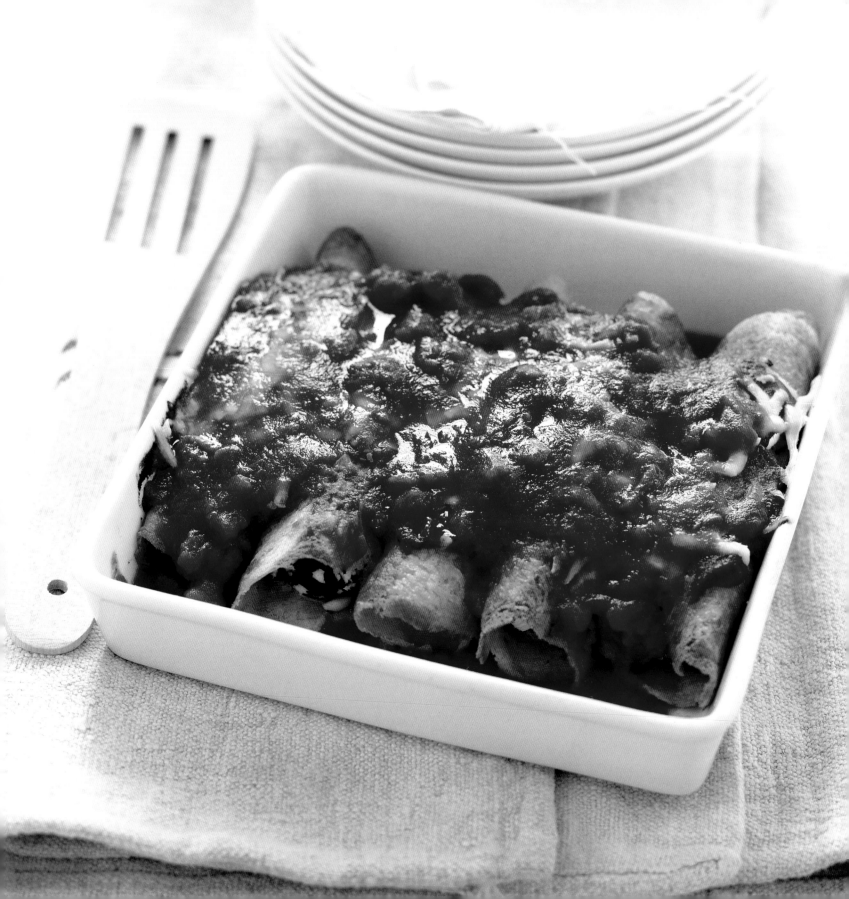

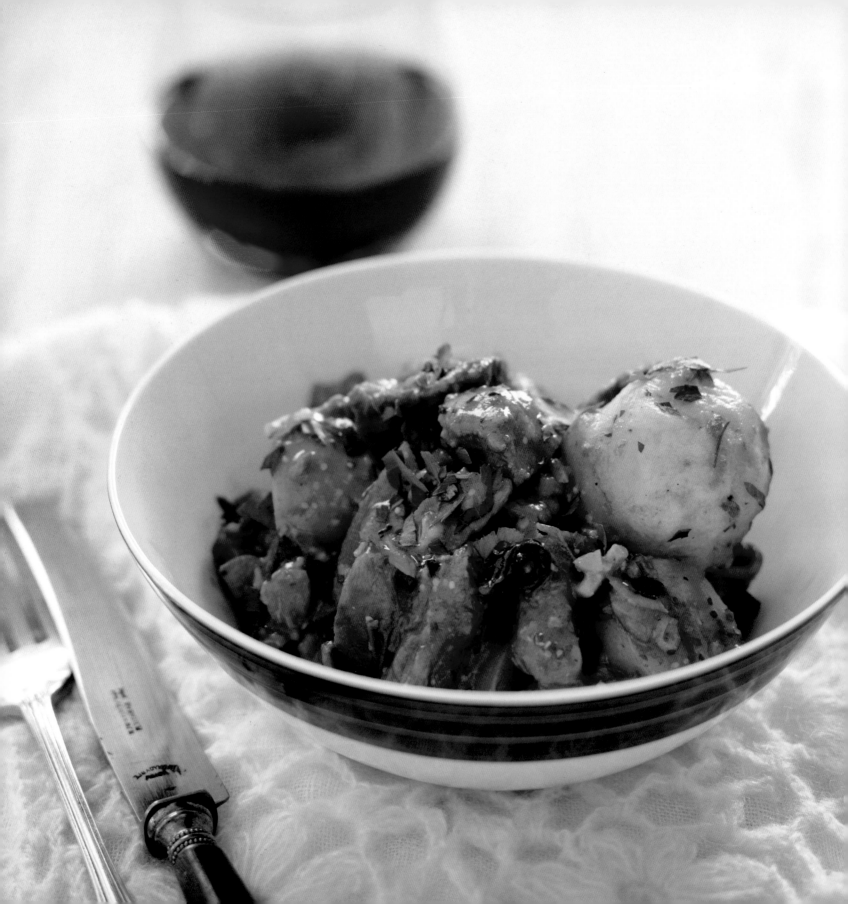

Beef and bacon casserole with dumplings

SERVES 6

Dumplings are an old-fashioned favourite, but because they are normally wheat-based they're off the menu for many people. Not any more. Now you can enjoy a comforting casserole with lots of gravy, topped with plump, wheat-free potato dumplings.

Preheat the oven to 140°C.

Place the cornflour in a large bowl and season with salt and pepper. Toss the beef in the seasoned flour, shaking off any excess.

Heat 2 tablespoons oil in a flameproof casserole dish over medium heat and cook the bacon and potato for 6–8 minutes or until the potato is golden and tender. Transfer the mixture to a bowl.

Heat 1 tablespoon oil in the casserole dish, add half the beef and cook, stirring occasionally, for 2 minutes or until browned all over. Transfer to a bowl. Repeat with the remaining oil and beef. Return the beef and the potato mixture to the dish.

Combine the brandy, mustard, cream and stock and pour into the dish. Bring to the boil over medium heat, then remove from the heat and season with salt and pepper. Cover and cook in the oven for 2 hours.

Meanwhile, to make the dumplings, place the potatoes in a large saucepan and cover with cold water. Bring to the boil and cook for 15 minutes or until tender when pierced with a skewer. Drain and set aside for 5 minutes to cool slightly then return to the pan. Add the milk and butter and mash with a potato masher until smooth. Sift the flours three times into a medium bowl (or mix well with a whisk to ensure they are well combined). Stir the sifted flours, cheese and parsley into the mash and season to taste with salt and pepper. Shape into 12 dumplings.

Remove the casserole dish from the oven, stir in the spinach and top with the dumplings. Cover and cook for 20 minutes, then remove the lid and cook for a further 15–20 minutes or until the dumplings are golden and the beef is very tender. Garnish with parsley and serve.

2 tablespoons maize cornflour

salt and freshly ground black pepper

1.2 kg boneless beef blade steak, cut into 3 cm cubes

⅓ cup (80 ml) garlic-infused canola oil

500 g lean bacon rashers, cut into thin strips

700 g chat potatoes, cut in half

½ cup (125 ml) brandy

2 tablespoons wholegrain mustard

½ cup (125 ml) reduced-fat cream

1 cup (250 ml) onion-free beef stock (gluten-free if on a gluten-free diet) (use more if required)

4 cups (80 g) baby spinach leaves

chopped flat-leaf parsley, to garnish

DUMPLINGS

2 large desiree potatoes, peeled

¾ cup (185 ml) low-fat milk

40 g butter

¾ cup (100 g) fine rice flour

½ cup (75 g) maize cornflour

3 tablespoons tapioca flour

½ cup (40 g) grated parmesan

2 tablespoons chopped flat-leaf parsley

salt and freshly ground black pepper

Pork ragout

SERVES 6

'Ragout' is the French name for a thick, rich stew that can be made with or without vegetables (this one does feature vegetables). It is delicious served with creamy mashed potato, but it is also great with rice or gluten-free pasta.

Heat 2 tablespoons oil in a large flameproof casserole dish over medium–high heat. Add the pork leg and cook for 2–3 minutes each side until browned all over. Remove the pork and set aside on a plate.

Heat the remaining oil in the dish, add the carrot, celery, bay leaves and sage and cook over medium–high heat for about 5 minutes until softened, stirring regularly. Add the stock, pureed tomato, potato and pork. Bring to the boil, then reduce the heat to low and simmer, covered, for 1½ hours or until the pork is tender. Turn the pork occasionally during cooking, and baste with the liquid. Remove the pork from the dish and rest on a plate.

Increase the heat to medium–high and bring the sauce to the boil. Simmer gently for 20 minutes or until thickened.

Cut the meat from the bone in large pieces and add to the sauce. Season with salt and pepper and serve with mashed potato, rice or gluten-free pasta.

3 tablespoons garlic-infused canola oil

1.5 kg pork leg, trimmed of fat

2 carrots, cut into small dice

2 stalks celery, cut into small dice

2 bay leaves

2 tablespoons chopped sage leaves

2 cups (500 ml) onion-free chicken stock (gluten-free if on a gluten-free diet)

700 ml pureed tomato

4 potatoes, cut into small dice

salt and freshly ground black pepper

mashed potato, rice or gluten-free pasta, to serve

Chicken with maple mustard sauce

SERVES 4

The unusual combination of maple syrup and mustard works brilliantly in this simple and delicious chicken dish.

Heat the oil in a large frying pan over medium–low heat and cook the chicken for 3–5 minutes each side, or until just cooked and golden brown. Remove from pan, then cover and leave to rest while you make the sauce.

For the sauce, combine the cornflour and a little chicken stock to form a paste. Gradually pour in the remaining stock, stirring well to ensure there are no lumps. Add the maple syrup, mustard, thyme, pepper and cream.

Pour the sauce into the frying pan and stir over medium–high heat for about 3–5 minutes or until the sauce thickens. Return the chicken pieces to the pan and toss through the sauce for 1–2 minutes to heat through. Season to taste, then serve immediately.

2 tablespoons garlic-infused canola oil

4 × 150 g skinless chicken breast fillets

MAPLE MUSTARD SAUCE

1 tablespoon maize cornflour

1 cup (250 ml) onion-free chicken stock
    (gluten-free if on a gluten-free diet)

3 tablespoons pure maple syrup

1 tablespoon wholegrain mustard

2 tablespoons chopped thyme

½ teaspoon freshly ground
    black pepper

2 tablespoons pouring cream

salt

Herbed beef meatballs with creamy potato nutmeg mash

SERVES 6

A winter favourite for the whole family. The gravy tastes great with an added splash of red wine, but feel free to leave it out to suit a younger palate.

To make the mash, place the potatoes in a large saucepan and cover with cold water. Bring to the boil and cook for 15 minutes or until tender when pierced with a skewer. Drain and set aside for 5 minutes to cool slightly. Peel the potatoes and return to the pan. Add the remaining ingredients and mash with a potato masher until smooth. Cover and keep warm.

Meanwhile, combine the beef, breadcrumbs, egg, oregano, marjoram and parsley in a large bowl. Season with salt and pepper. Roll the mixture into walnut-sized balls.

Heat a little oil in a large heavy-based frying pan over medium heat and cook the meatballs for 6–8 minutes or until browned and cooked through.

To make the gravy, combine all the ingredients in a small bowl and stir well to form a paste. Slowly add 1 cup (250 ml) boiling water, stirring constantly to ensure there are no lumps and the gravy thickens evenly.

Divide the mash among six plates and top with the meatballs. Spoon the gravy over the meatballs and serve, garnished with the extra oregano.

600 g lean minced beef
½ cup (50 g) dried gluten-free breadcrumbs
3 eggs, lightly beaten
2 tablespoons chopped oregano, plus extra leaves to garnish
2 tablespoons chopped marjoram
⅓ cup (10 g) chopped flat-leaf parsley
salt and freshly ground black pepper
canola oil, for pan-frying

CREAMY POTATO NUTMEG MASH
6 large sebago or coliban potatoes
½ cup (125 ml) milk
60 g butter
pinch of salt
⅓ cup (40 g) coarsely grated cheddar
pinch of ground nutmeg

TOMATO GRAVY
3 tablespoons onion-free gravy powder (gluten-free if on a gluten-free diet)
2 tablespoons tomato paste (puree)
2 tablespoons dry red wine (optional)

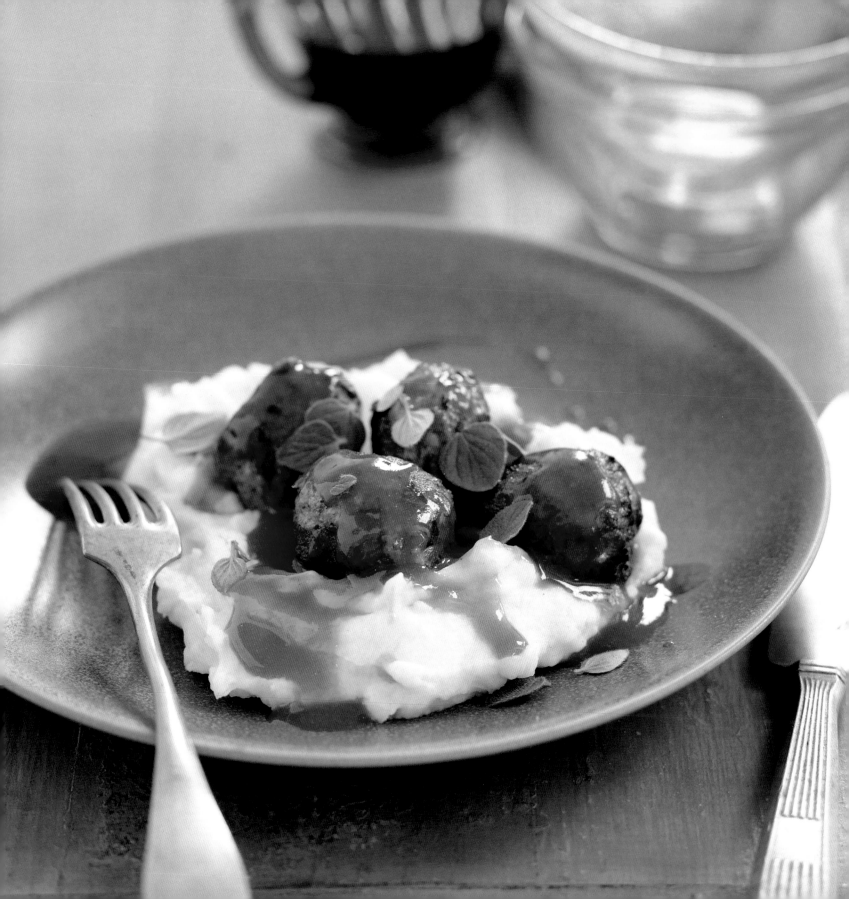

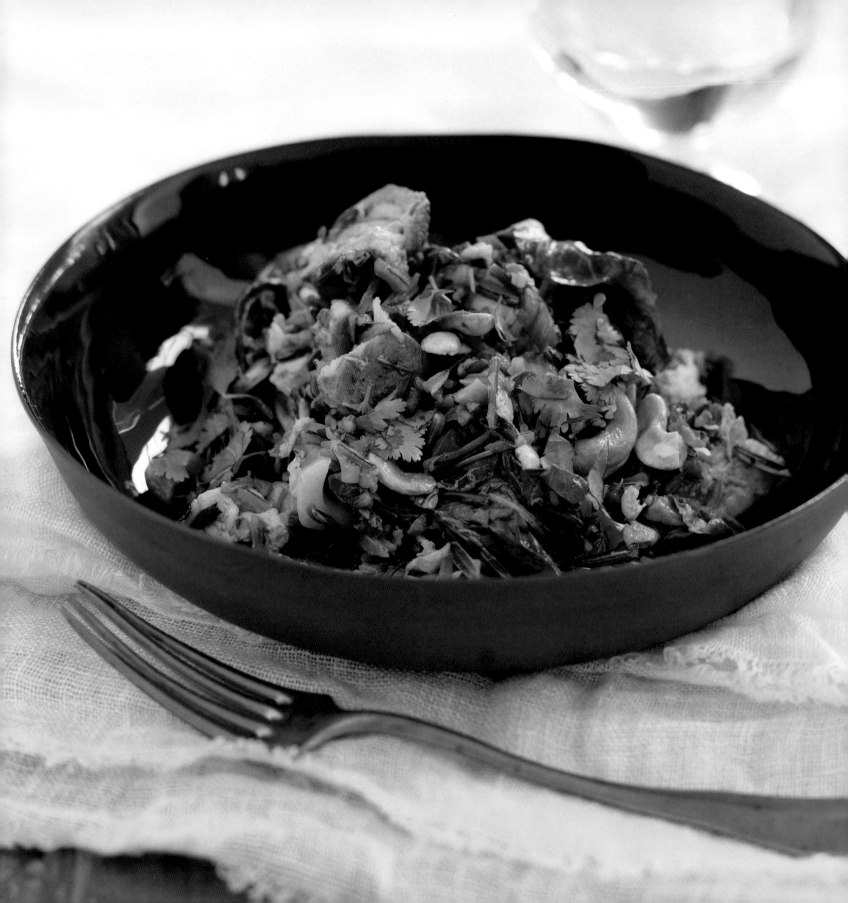

Chinese chicken on fried wild rice

SERVES 4

Wild rice looks and tastes sensational, and makes a nice change from regular white rice. Here, its distinctive nutty flavour is enhanced by a handful of roasted cashews.

Combine the soy sauce, ginger, oil and five-spice powder in a jug. Place the chicken fillets in a non-metallic dish, pour the marinade over the top and toss to coat. Cover and marinate in the fridge for 2–3 hours.

To start preparing the fried rice, place the rice in a medium saucepan and cover with 900 ml cold water. Bring to the boil and cook, covered, over medium heat for 45 minutes or until tender and beginning to curl. Drain and set aside for 20 minutes.

Preheat the oven to 180°C.

Place the chicken in a large non-stick frying pan and cook over medium–high heat for 2 minutes each side. Transfer to a roasting tin and bake for about 20–25 minutes or until cooked through, turning once. Remove from the oven and set aside in a warm place.

Meanwhile, to make the fried rice, heat 1 teaspoon oil in a large frying pan and cook the cashews, stirring frequently, until lightly toasted. Transfer to a plate. Heat the remaining oil in the pan and cook the egg, stirring and breaking it up into pieces. Add the rice, cashews and soy sauce and cook, stirring regularly, for 2–3 minutes until heated through. Remove from the heat, stir in the coriander and season to taste.

Cut the chicken into 1 cm thick slices and toss through the fried rice. Divide among four plates, garnish with the extra coriander and serve immediately with steamed Asian greens.

3 tablespoons soy sauce (gluten-free
   if on a gluten-free diet)
2 teaspoons grated ginger
1 tablespoon garlic-infused canola oil
1 teaspoon Chinese five-spice powder
4 × 200 g skinless chicken breast fillets
steamed Asian greens, to serve

FRIED WILD RICE
200 g wild rice
2 teaspoons peanut oil
½ cup (75 g) roasted cashews,
   roughly chopped
2 eggs, lightly beaten
1 tablespoon soy sauce (gluten-free
   if on a gluten-free diet)
2 tablespoons coarsely chopped
   coriander, plus extra to garnish
salt and freshly ground black pepper

Peppered lamb with rosemary cottage potatoes

SERVES 6

The key to serving juicy, tender roast meat is to let it rest before you slice it. This is because the fibres in the meat tighten during cooking, and the resting process allows them to relax. In this recipe, the lamb rests while the cottage potatoes are cooking.

Place the lamb in a roasting tin. Rub with pepper, then cover with plastic film and refrigerate for 3–4 hours.

Preheat the oven to 200°C.

Roast the lamb for 1 hour 20 minutes for medium, or to taste.

Meanwhile, to make the cottage potatoes, place the potatoes in a large saucepan of cold water. Bring to the boil and cook for 10–12 minutes or until tender. Drain and cool, then peel and cut in half. Combine the potato and cheese in a large bowl and season with salt and pepper. Transfer to a medium baking dish.

Place the butter and rosemary in a small frying pan over medium heat and stir until the butter is melted and lightly golden. Pour over the potato mixture, followed by the milk.

As soon as the lamb is ready, remove it from the roasting tin and transfer to a plate. Cover with foil and leave to rest. Place the cottage potatoes in the oven and bake for 20–25 minutes.

While the potatoes are baking, place the lamb roasting tin over medium heat, add the wine and cook for 5 minutes or until reduced by half. Add the stock and bring to the boil. Reduce the heat and simmer, stirring regularly, for 5 minutes or until the sauce starts to thicken. Remove the tin from the heat and stir in the sour cream until melted and well combined. Season with salt and pepper.

Carve the lamb and serve with the red wine sauce, cottage potatoes and steamed vegetables on the side.

1.5 kg lamb leg roast
2 tablespoons freshly ground
    black pepper
½ cup (125 ml) dry red wine
1 cup (250 ml) onion-free beef stock
    (gluten-free if on a gluten-free diet)
3 tablespoons sour cream
salt and freshly ground black pepper
steamed vegetables, to serve

ROSEMARY COTTAGE POTATOES

10 small potatoes
200 g cheddar, cut into cubes
salt and freshly ground black pepper
50 g butter
2 tablespoons rosemary leaves
½ cup (125 ml) low-fat milk

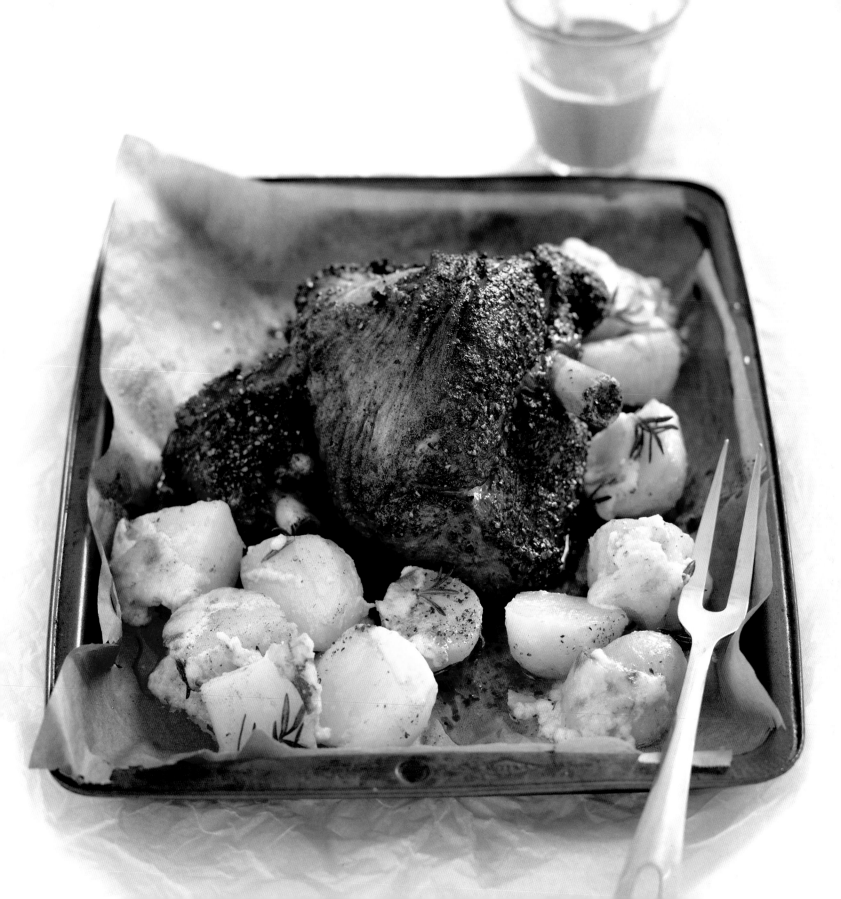

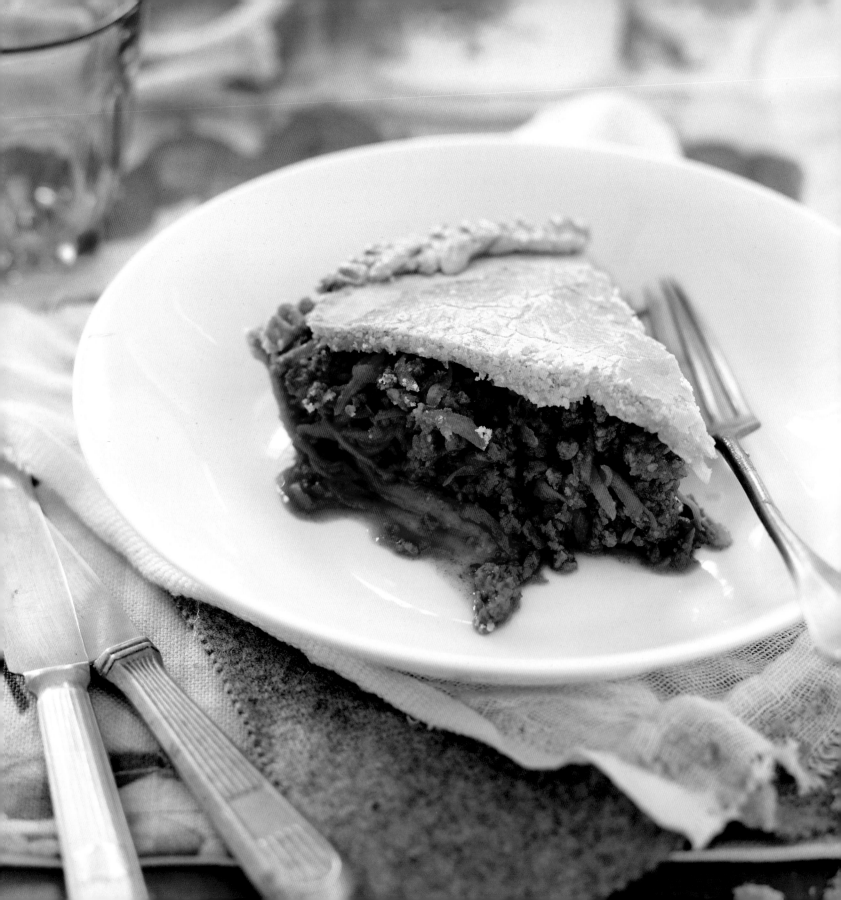

Family beef pie

SERVES 4

Most meat pies contain wheat pastry and onion, making them unsuitable for people following the Low-FODMAP Diet. This doesn't seem fair so I've come up with a recipe the whole family can enjoy. The amount of soy flour used in this recipe is minimal so it will suit most people following the Low-FODMAP Diet. Assess your individual tolerance.

To make the pastry, sift the flours and xanthan gum three times into a bowl (or mix well with a whisk to ensure they are well combined). Transfer to a food processor, add the butter and process until the mixture resembles fine breadcrumbs. While the motor is running, add the iced water (a tablespoon at a time) to form a soft dough. You may not need all the water. Turn out onto a bench dusted with gluten-free cornflour and knead until smooth. Divide the dough into two portions, wrap in plastic film and refrigerate for 30 minutes.

Preheat the oven to 170°C. Grease a shallow 18 cm pie tin.

Place one portion of dough between two sheets of baking paper and roll out to a thickness of 3–5 mm. Invert the pie tin on the pastry and, using a small sharp knife, cut out a circle of pastry. Set aside (this will be the top). Roll out the remaining piece of dough and cut out another circle of pastry – but this time allow an extra 1 cm from the tin edge. This will be the pie base. Ease the pastry base into the tin and trim the edges to neaten.

Line the pastry case with baking paper, fill with baking beads or rice and blind-bake for 10–15 minutes or until lightly golden. Remove the baking paper and beads or rice and set aside to cool.

To make the filling, brown the minced beef in a non-stick saucepan over medium heat. Add the carrot, gravy powder, soy sauce and 1½ cups (375 ml) water and cook for 8–10 minutes or until the mixture forms a thick gravy.

Spoon the filling into the cooled pie base. Brush a little beaten egg on the pastry edge, then place the pastry lid on top, pressing gently to seal. Brush the top with beaten egg and bake for 20–25 minutes or until golden brown.

800 g lean minced beef

2 carrots, grated

100 g onion-free gravy powder
(gluten-free if on a gluten-free diet)

1 teaspoon gluten-free soy sauce

1 egg, lightly beaten

PASTRY

1 cup (130 g) fine rice flour

½ cup (75 g) maize cornflour

½ cup (45 g) debittered soy flour

1 teaspoon xanthan gum

160 g butter, chopped

80–120 ml iced water

Roast pork with chestnut stuffing

SERVES 8

Chestnut meal is made from coarsely ground chestnuts, and is often sold frozen. It may be hard to find in supermarkets, so your best bet is to look for it in gourmet delis. Use it in soups, cakes and crumbles or, as in this recipe, as a base for stuffing. If you can't find any, natural almond meal may be used instead.

Preheat the oven to 220°C.

Combine the chestnut meal, breadcrumbs, herbs and brown sugar in a bowl. Season with salt and pepper, then stir in the balsamic vinegar.

Open out the pork and spoon the stuffing down the centre. Roll up the pork to enclose the filling and tie with kitchen string at 2 cm intervals.

Transfer the pork to a roasting tin and roast for 25 minutes. Reduce the temperature to 190°C and cook for a further hour. Remove the pork to a plate, then cover with foil and rest for 20 minutes. Cut into slices and serve with roast vegetables (such as potato, carrot and parsnip) and steamed zucchini flowers, garnished with the extra sage leaves.

100 g chestnut meal

1½ cups (110 g) fresh gluten-free breadcrumbs (made from day-old bread)

⅓ cup (10 g) chopped flat-leaf parsley

2 tablespoons chopped sage leaves, plus extra leaves to garnish

3 tablespoons brown sugar

salt and freshly ground black pepper

3 tablespoons balsamic vinegar

2 kg boned rolled pork loin with crackling

roast vegetables and steamed zucchini (courgette) flowers, to serve

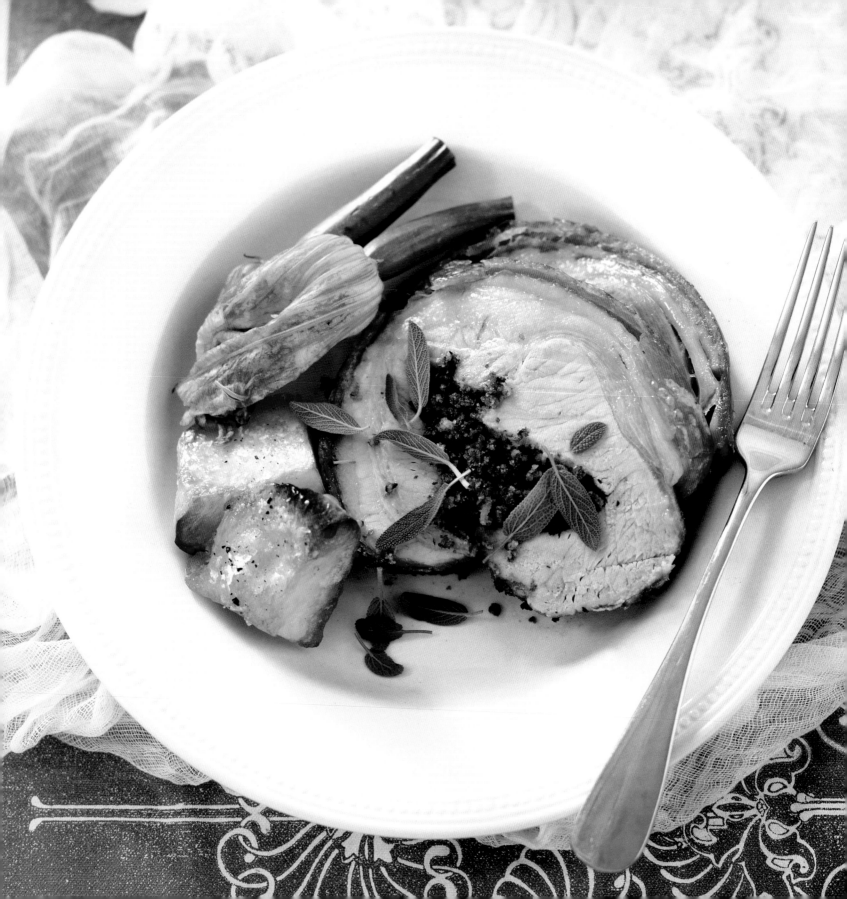

Chicken and capsicum pilau

SERVES 6–8

I love the versatility of rice – it fits right in with so many different styles of cooking. A pilau (also called pilaf) involves heating the rice in oil and then cooking it gently in a stock or broth.

Rinse the rice under cold water until the water runs clear. Place the rice in a bowl, cover with cold water and leave to soak for 20 minutes.

Combine the saffron and 1 tablespoon hot water in a cup, then set aside to infuse.

Heat 2 tablespoons oil in a large frying pan over medium–high heat and cook the chicken and celery, stirring regularly, for 5–6 minutes or until the chicken is golden brown and the celery has softened. Transfer to a plate.

Reduce the heat to medium–low, add the remaining oil, cinnamon, cardamom, cloves, star anise, curry leaves, ginger and chilli to the pan and cook, stirring, for 1 minute or until fragrant. Drain the rice and add to the pan, stirring to coat well in the spice mixture.

Increase the heat to high and add the saffron mixture, stock and chicken. Bring to the boil, then reduce the heat to low and cook, covered, for 20 minutes or until the rice is tender and the liquid has been absorbed. Remove from the heat and stir in the sliced capsicum. Cover and set aside for about 10 minutes before serving.

2 cups (400 g) basmati rice

small pinch of saffron threads

3 tablespoons garlic-infused canola oil

750 g skinless chicken breast fillets, sliced

2 stalks celery, cut into thin slices

3 cm piece cinnamon stick

2 green cardamom pods

2 cloves

1 star anise

20 fresh curry leaves

1 tablespoon chopped ginger

2 small red chillies, finely chopped

3 cups (750 ml) onion-free chicken stock (gluten-free if on a gluten-free diet)

½ red capsicum (pepper), sliced

½ green capsicum (pepper), sliced

½ yellow capsicum (pepper), sliced

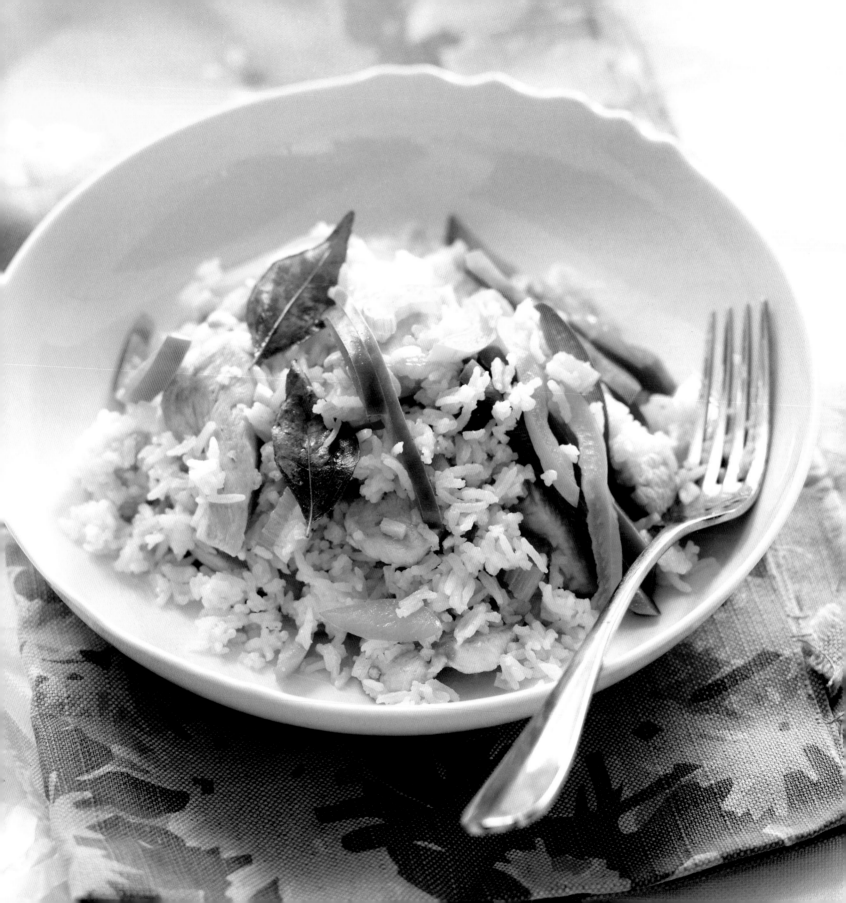

Dukkah-crusted barramundi

SERVES 4

Dukkah is an Egyptian spice blend typically made with sesame seeds, nuts, ground coriander and cumin. I like to serve these cutlets with gently spiced rice, made by stirring a little butter, ½ teaspoon ground cumin and 1 tablespoon finely chopped coriander through steamed rice, but plain rice is also delicious.

To make the dukkah, preheat the oven to 180°C and line a baking tray with baking paper. Spread out the almonds and pine nuts on the tray and bake for 5 minutes or until golden. Cool to room temperature. Place all the nuts and spices in a food processor and process until fine crumbs are formed. Reserve 4 tablespoons to serve and transfer the rest to a plate.

 Brush the barramundi cutlets with a little oil, then press into the dukkah to coat both sides. Heat a chargrill pan over medium–high heat. Add the fish and cook for 3–4 minutes each side or until just cooked. Sprinkle with coriander and the reserved dukkah and serve with rice and lemon wedges.

4 × 200 g barramundi cutlets
 (ideally about 3 cm thick)
2 tablespoons canola oil
coriander leaves, to serve
steamed rice, to serve
lemon wedges, to serve

DUKKAH

150 g blanched almonds
60 g pine nuts
1 teaspoon ground coriander
1 teaspoon cumin seeds
1 teaspoon sesame seeds
½ teaspoon chilli powder

Tuscan tuna pasta

SERVES 4

These days, there are so many varieties of gluten-free pasta available that you can enjoy this simple dish with any shaped pasta you like.

Combine the oil, chilli and tomatoes in a jar and shake well to combine. Set aside for 1 hour.

 Cook the pasta in a large saucepan of boiling water until just tender. Drain and return to the pan. Stir in the oil mixture, tuna, olives and half the basil.

 Divide among four bowls and top with the parmesan and remaining basil.

3 tablespoons garlic-infused olive oil
1 teaspoon dried chilli flakes
100 g semi-dried tomatoes, chopped
500 g gluten-free pasta
200 g tinned tuna, drained and flaked
½ cup (80 g) chopped kalamata olives
½ cup (30 g) shredded basil
½ cup (40 g) grated parmesan

Dukkah-crusted barramundi →

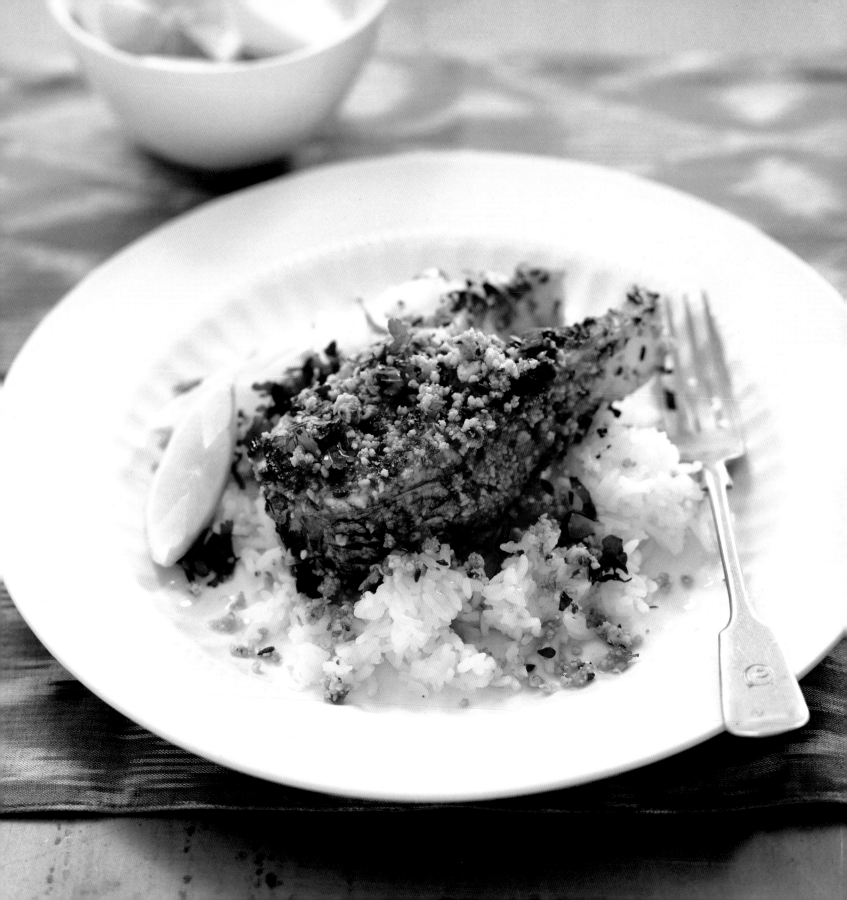

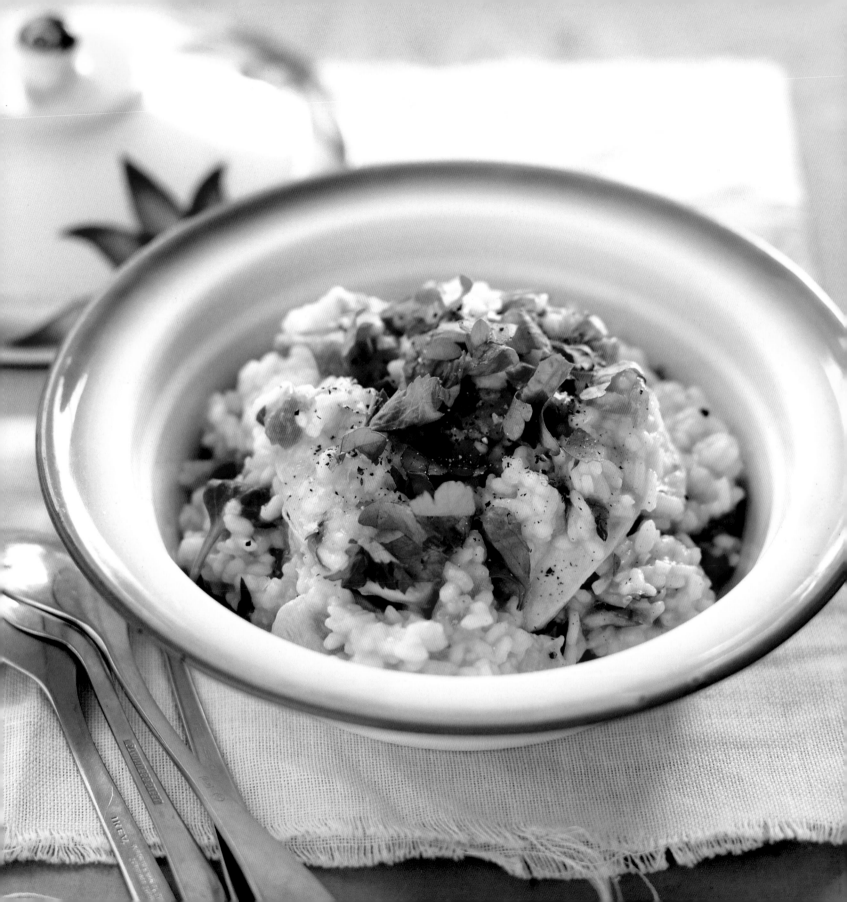

Tomato chicken risotto

SERVES 6

There's something very comforting about a bowl of creamy risotto, especially when it's homemade. This version is free of onions and garlic so it is suitable for people following the Low-FODMAP Diet.

Heat 1 tablespoon oil in a small frying pan over medium–high heat and cook the chicken until just cooked and lightly golden, tossing regularly. Remove and set aside.

Pour the stock into a saucepan over low heat and keep at a low simmer.

Heat the remaining oil in a large heavy-based saucepan, add the rice and stir for 1–2 minutes until the rice is well coated with oil. Pour in the wine and cook until absorbed. Add 1 cup (250 ml) stock and cook, stirring, until absorbed. Add the remaining stock ½ cup (125 ml) at a time, reserving the last ½ cup (125 ml) stock for later.

Add the chicken, spinach, tinned tomatoes, parmesan and parsley and stir until well combined. Pour in the reserved stock, stirring until completely absorbed. Season with salt and pepper and serve garnished with extra parsley leaves.

2 tablespoons garlic-infused olive oil

400 g skinless chicken breast fillets, sliced

2 litres onion-free chicken stock (gluten-free if on a gluten-free diet)

2½ cups (500 g) arborio rice

½ cup (125 ml) white wine

2 cups (40 g) baby spinach leaves

220 g tinned chopped tomatoes

½ cup (40 g) grated parmesan

3 tablespoons chopped flat-leaf parsley, plus extra leaves to garnish

salt and freshly ground black pepper

Risotto Milanese

SERVES 6

This simple, traditionally flavoured risotto may be enjoyed as is, but its mild flavour also makes it a perfect base for meat and poultry dishes. I particularly like it with slow-cooked meat, so tender it's falling off the bone.

Heat the oil in a large saucepan, add the saffron and stir over medium heat for 2 minutes. Add the rice and stir for 1–2 minutes or until the rice is well coated in the oil and saffron mixture.

Pour the stock into a medium saucepan over low heat and keep at a low simmer.

Add the wine to the rice and cook until absorbed. Pour in 1 cup (250 ml) stock and cook, stirring, until completely absorbed. Add the remaining stock ½ cup (125 ml) at a time, reserving the last ½ cup (125 ml) stock for later.

Stir in the parmesan and parsley. Pour in the reserved stock, stirring until completely absorbed. Taste, season with salt and pepper and serve.

1 tablespoon garlic-infused olive oil
1 teaspoon saffron threads
2½ cups (500 g) arborio rice
2 litres onion-free vegetable stock
(gluten-free if on a gluten-free diet)
½ cup (125 ml) white wine
½ cup (40 g) grated parmesan
3 tablespoons chopped flat-leaf parsley
salt and freshly ground black pepper

Balsamic sesame swordfish

SERVES 4

Swordfish is a meaty fish, purchased as steaks, so there is no wastage. If you can't find it, this recipe also works very well with tuna steaks.

Combine the balsamic vinegar, soy sauce and brown sugar in a non-metallic bowl. Add the swordfish steaks and toss to coat in the marinade, then cover and refrigerate for 3–4 hours, turning regularly.

Preheat the oven to 230°C. Line a large baking tray with baking paper.

Place the swordfish steaks on the tray, reserving the marinade, and bake for 10 minutes. Turn the steaks over and baste with the marinade. Sprinkle with sesame seeds and bake for a further 5–10 minutes or until cooked through. Serve with steamed Asian greens.

3 tablespoons balsamic vinegar

2 tablespoons soy sauce (gluten-free if on a gluten-free diet)

2 tablespoons brown sugar

4 large swordfish steaks

1½ tablespoons sesame seeds

steamed Asian greens, to serve

Thai-inspired stir-fry with tofu and vermicelli noodles

SERVES 4

Many noodles, such as hokkien, udon and egg noodles, are made from wheat and are therefore not suitable for people on the Low-FODMAP Diet. However, all is not lost: rice vermicelli noodles are available in a range of thicknesses, or try glass noodles (made from mungbeans) or 100% buckwheat soba noodles. Tofu is a great vegetarian protein source that is tolerated by many on the Low-FODMAP Diet. Assess your individual tolerance.

Soak the noodles in boiling water until soft. Drain and set aside.

Combine the sweet chilli sauce, fish sauce and ginger in a small bowl.

In a cup, blend a little warm water into the cornflour to form a paste, then add the remaining water and mix well. Pour this into the sweet chilli sauce mixture and mix with a metal spoon until well combined.

Heat the oil in a medium frying pan over medium–high heat, add the tofu and cook, turning once, for 3 minutes or until golden brown. Add the sauce and stir gently until the sauce thickens. Stir in the noodles, coriander and mint and serve immediately, garnished with the crushed peanuts.

250 g rice vermicelli noodles
⅔ cup (160 ml) sweet chilli sauce
2 tablespoons fish sauce
2 teaspoons grated ginger
1 cup (250 ml) warm water
1 tablespoon maize cornflour
1 tablespoon garlic-infused peanut oil
500 g firm tofu, cut into thick slices
4 tablespoons chopped coriander
1 cup (50 g) chopped mint
2 tablespoons crushed peanuts

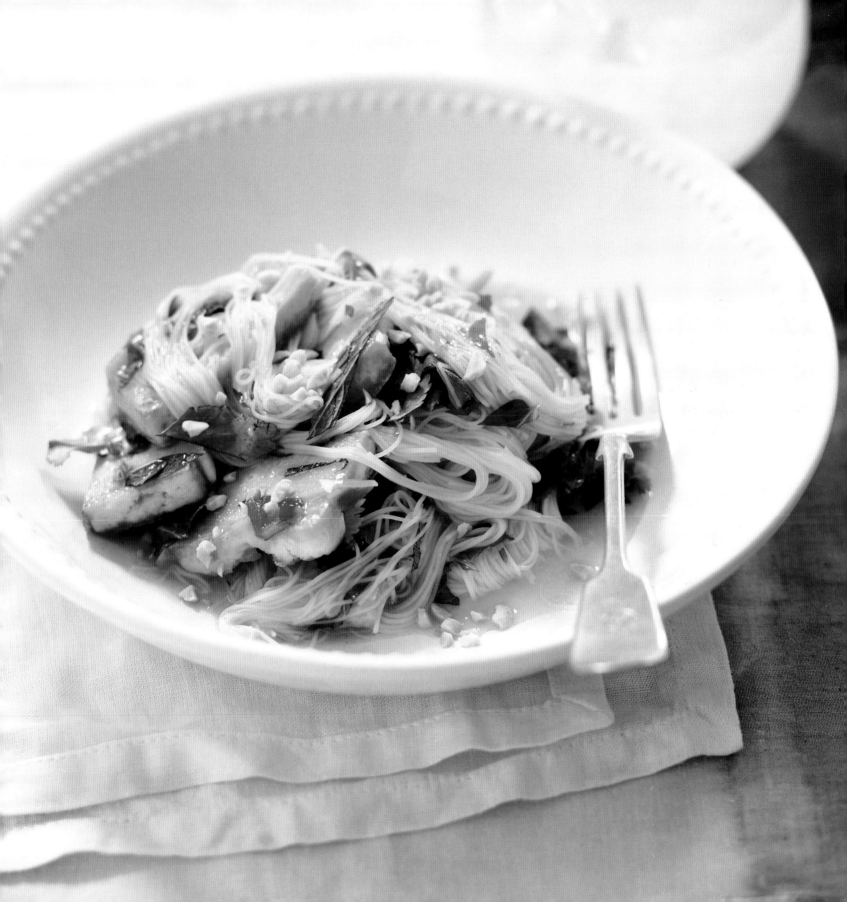

Stir-fried kangaroo with chilli and coriander

SERVES 4

Kangaroo is a nutritious, lean meat with a slightly gamey flavour that is becoming increasingly popular – in fact, most larger supermarkets now stock it. It can dry out quickly because it is so lean, so take care not to overcook it.

Place the chilli, sherry, cornflour and brown sugar in a small jar and shake to combine well.

Heat 1 teaspoon oil in a large wok or frying pan over high heat, add half the kangaroo strips and toss until just cooked. Remove and transfer to a plate. Repeat with the remaining kangaroo strips.

Heat the remaining oil in the wok or pan and stir-fry the carrot and celery for 3 minutes or until tender but starting to crisp around the edges. Add the chilli mixture and kangaroo strips and stir-fry for another 2 minutes. Remove from the heat, stir in the coriander and serve immediately with steamed rice.

1 small red chilli, thinly sliced

2 tablespoons dry sherry

2 teaspoons maize cornflour

2 teaspoons brown sugar

2 teaspoons sesame oil

500 g kangaroo rump steak, cut into thin strips

2 carrots, finely sliced on the diagonal

2 stalks celery, finely sliced on the diagonal

⅓ cup (20 g) coriander leaves

steamed rice, to serve

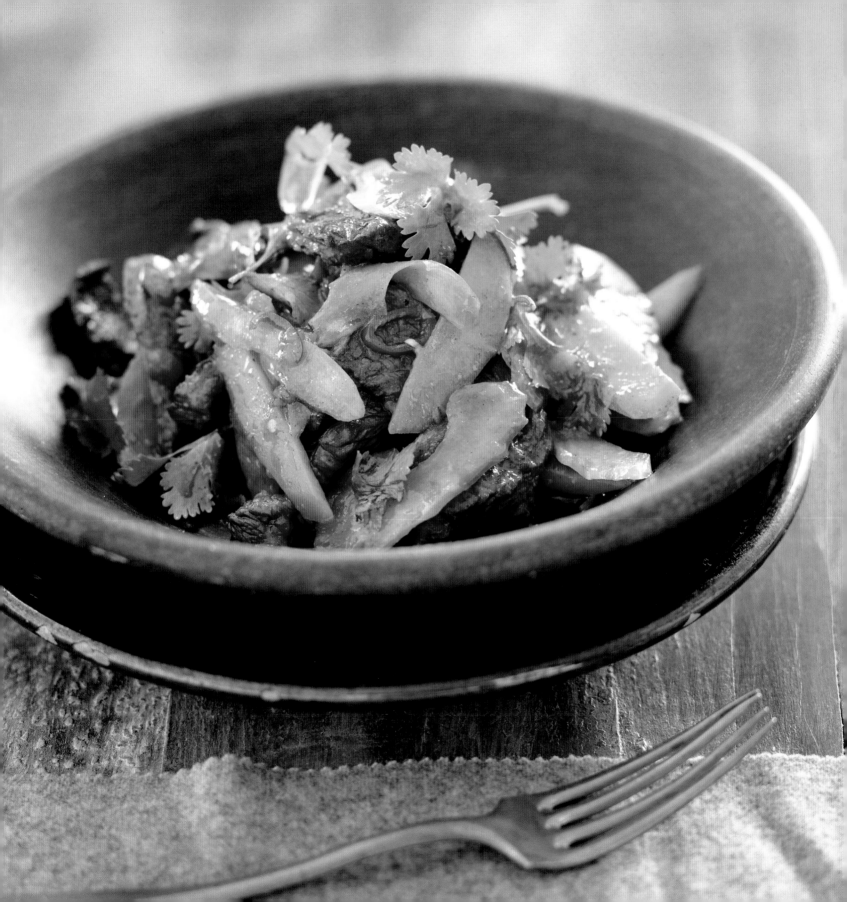

Spinach and pancetta pasta

SERVES 4

Pancetta is unsmoked dried pork belly that has been salt cured and spiced. It may be eaten raw but is often lightly pan-fried to enhance its depth of flavour – I find this makes a big difference, especially in simple dishes like this one.

Cook the pasta in a large saucepan of boiling water until just tender. Drain and return to the pan. Stir in 2 tablespoons oil, then cover to keep warm.

Heat the remaining oil in a large frying pan and cook the pancetta, spinach and pine nuts until the pine nuts are golden and the spinach has wilted. Add the pasta and parmesan and toss over medium heat until the cheese has melted. Season to taste with salt and pepper and serve with an extra splash of oil, if desired.

500 g gluten-free pasta
3 tablespoons garlic-infused olive oil, plus extra to serve (optional)
200 g thinly sliced pancetta
100 g baby spinach leaves
⅓ cup (50 g) pine nuts
½ cup (40 g) grated parmesan
salt and freshly ground black pepper

Pasta with ricotta and lemon

SERVES 4

People with lactose intolerance can still enjoy this delicious pasta dish – simply replace the fresh ricotta with shredded buffalo mozzarella or bocconcini. It won't melt through in quite the same way as ricotta, but will still result in a most enjoyable meal.

Cook the pasta in a large saucepan of boiling water until just tender. Drain and return to the pan.

Combine the ricotta, spinach, parsley, lemon zest and lemon juice in a bowl then stir through the hot pasta. Season to taste. Garnish with the extra lemon zest if desired and serve immediately.

500 g gluten-free pasta
¾ cup (150 g) fresh ricotta
3 cups (60 g) baby spinach leaves
3 tablespoons chopped flat-leaf parsley
grated zest of 1 lemon
3 tablespoons lemon juice
salt and freshly ground black pepper
thin strips of lemon zest, extra, to serve (optional)

Spinach and pancetta pasta →

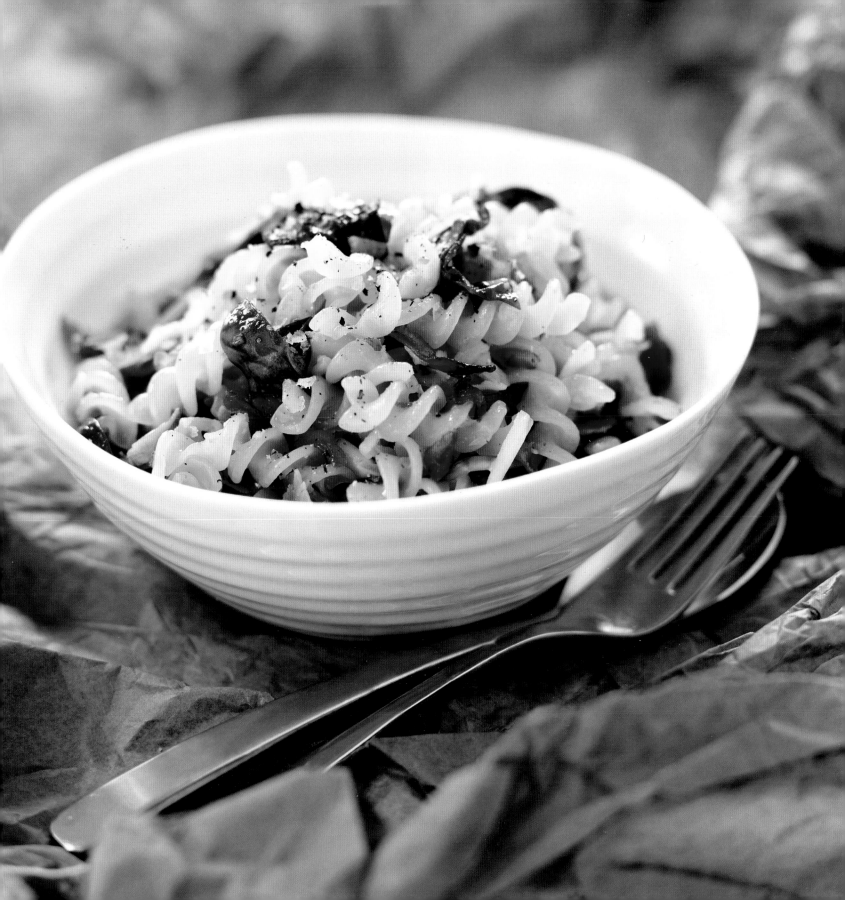

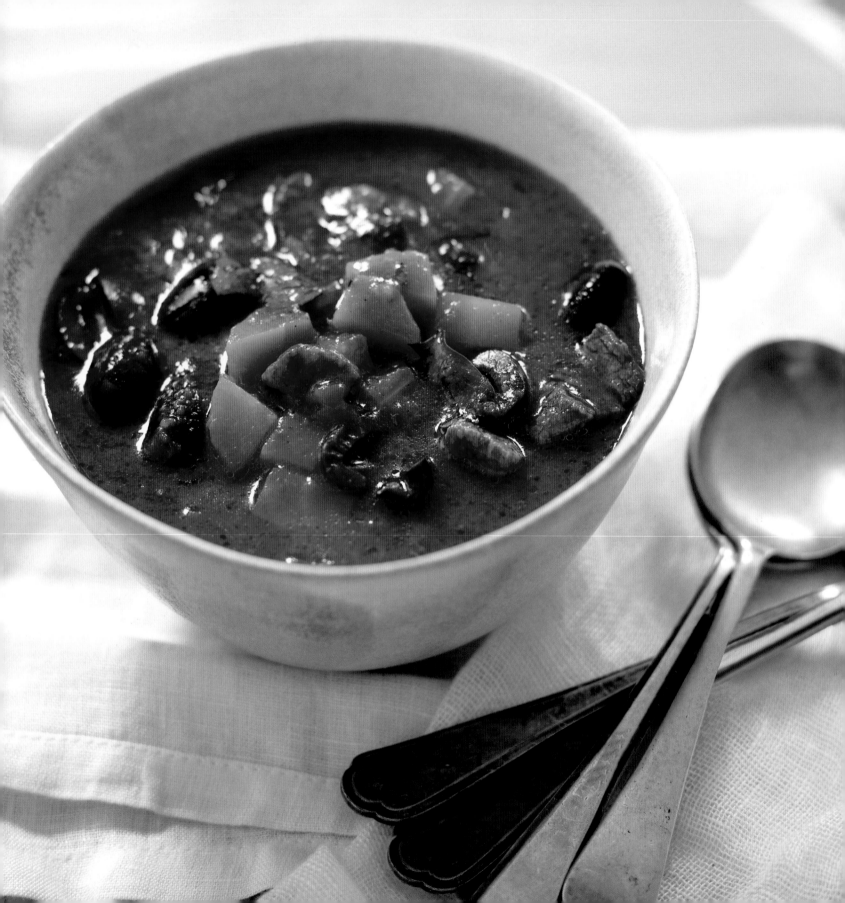

Warming winter beef soup

SERVES 4–6

This soup is full of flavour surprises – olives, orange zest, allspice . . .
But fear not: this unusual combination of ingredients works in perfect
harmony to create a very different soup that you are sure to enjoy.

Place the flour in a large bowl and season with salt and pepper. Add the beef
and toss to coat.

Heat 1 tablespoon oil in a large heavy-based saucepan or stockpot over
medium–low heat and cook the carrot and celery for 6–8 minutes until
softened and golden. Remove and set aside on a plate.

Heat 1 tablespoon oil in the pan and add half the beef. Toss until browned
on all sides then transfer to the plate with the vegetables. Repeat with the
remaining oil and beef.

Return the beef and vegetables to the pan. Increase the heat to medium–high
and pour in the wine, stock and pureed tomato. Stir through well, scraping up
any bits of meat caught on the base of the pan. Add the orange zest, allspice and
chilli flakes. Bring to the boil, then reduce the heat to medium–low and simmer
for 1 hour, stirring regularly.

Stir in the olives and parsley, season to taste and serve.

40 g maize cornflour

salt and freshly ground black pepper

800 g gravy beef or casserole steak,
    cut into 1 cm cubes

3 tablespoons vegetable oil

2 large carrots, diced

2 large stalks celery, diced

1 cup (250 ml) dry red wine

3 cups (750 ml) onion-free beef stock
    (gluten-free if on a gluten-free diet)

1½ cups (420 ml) pureed tomato

2 teaspoons finely grated orange zest

¼ teaspoon ground allspice

¼ teaspoon dried chilli flakes

100 g pitted kalamata olives, sliced

⅓ cup (10 g) chopped flat-leaf parsley

salt and freshly ground black pepper.

French veal with herb rosti

SERVES 4

Rosti are Swiss potato cakes with a crisp golden crust. They work best when the cooked potatoes are left to cool completely. This recipe makes four individual rosti, however one large one can be made by cooking the mixture in a medium frying pan.

Place the tarragon, oil, pepper and cornflour in a small screw-top jar and shake well to combine. Brush over the veal steaks, then cover and refrigerate for 1–2 hours.

To make the rosti, place the unpeeled potatoes in a large saucepan, cover with cold water and bring to the boil. Reduce the heat and simmer rapidly for 10 minutes. Drain, then set aside to cool.

Peel the potatoes, then grate the flesh into a large bowl. Add the herbs and melted butter and season to taste. Divide the mixture into four equal portions. Form each portion into a ball, then gently press flat with your hand.

Heat the oil in a large non-stick frying pan over medium heat. Add the rosti and cook for 10–15 minutes or until the base is crisp and golden. Flip with a spatula and cook for a further 10 minutes or until cooked through and the base is golden brown.

Heat a large non-stick frying pan over high heat and cook the steaks for about 3–4 minutes each side, or until cooked to your liking. Set aside to rest for a few minutes.

Return the pan to medium–high heat, add the red wine and stock and bring to a simmer. Add the veal steaks and heat through for 2 minutes. Serve immediately with the herb rosti, steamed carrots and a spoonful of mustard.

1 tablespoon finely chopped tarragon
1 tablespoon olive oil
2 tablespoons freshly ground
   black pepper
2 teaspoons maize cornflour
4 × 200 g veal steaks
⅓ cup (80 ml) red wine
½ cup (125 ml) onion-free beef stock
   (gluten-free if on a gluten-free diet)
steamed baby carrots, to serve
wholegrain mustard, to serve

HERB ROSTI

4 large pontiac potatoes
2 tablespoons chopped flat-leaf parsley
6 sage leaves, chopped
100 g butter, melted
salt and freshly ground black pepper
2 tablespoons vegetable oil

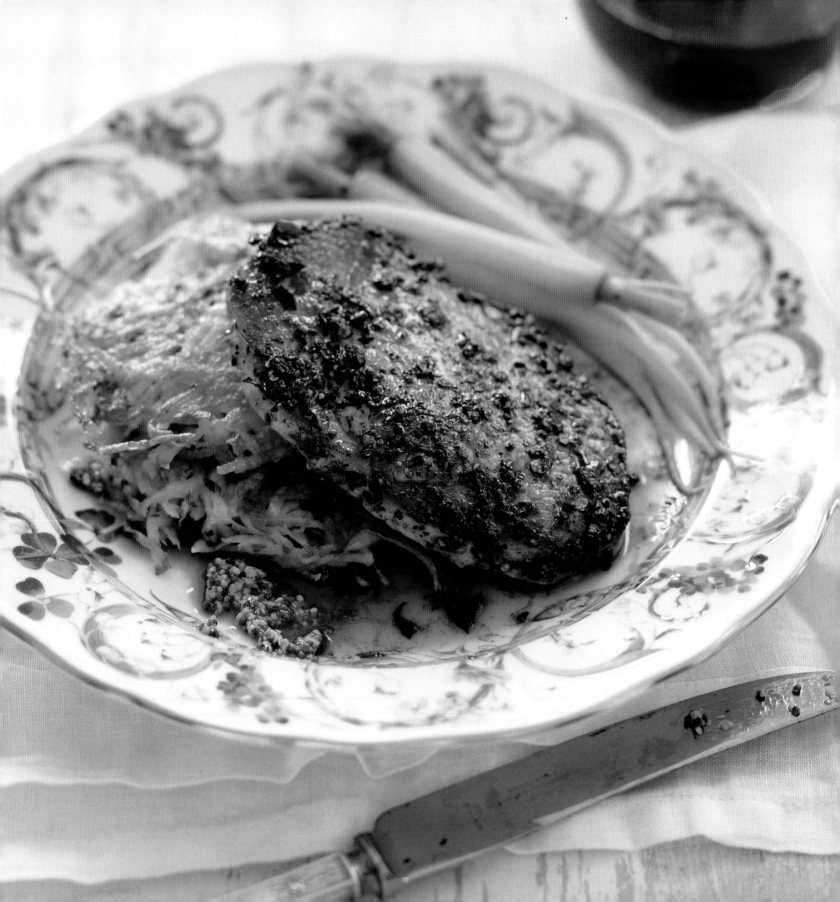

Paprika calamari with garden salad

SERVES 4

Calamari looks so inviting to eat when it is curled up, as it is in this recipe. The trick is to use thick pieces of squid. Cut them open, then with the inside of the squid facing up, cut in a criss-cross pattern. This will ensure the calamari curls beautifully during cooking.

Cut the squid hoods down the long sides to make two large pieces (if using large squid, cut them into quarters). With a sharp knife, cut the squid pieces in a 1 cm criss-cross pattern, taking care not to cut all the way through. Pat dry with paper towel.

Combine the salt, pepper, paprika and cornflour in a large bowl, add the squid pieces and toss to coat. Cover and refrigerate for 3–4 hours.

To prepare the salad, combine all the ingredients in a large salad bowl.

For the dressing, place all the ingredients in a small screw-top jar and shake well to combine.

Preheat a barbecue to hot, or heat a frying pan or chargrill pan over high heat. Brush with oil. Add the squid pieces, scored-side down, and cook for 2–3 minutes, then turn and cook for another 1–2 minutes.

Divide the salad among four bowls or plates and drizzle with the dressing. Arrange the paprika calamari on top and serve warm.

4 large or 8 regular squid hoods, cleaned
½ teaspoon salt
½ teaspoon finely ground black pepper
1 teaspoon paprika
⅓ cup (50 g) maize cornflour
olive oil, for cooking

GARDEN SALAD

1 baby cos lettuce, roughly chopped
½ large cucumber, halved lengthways and sliced
2 stalks celery, thinly sliced
½ green capsicum (pepper), seeded and sliced
1 cup (50 g) snowpea sprouts

DRESSING

3 tablespoons garlic-infused olive oil
1½ tablespoons lemon juice
½ teaspoon brown sugar
salt

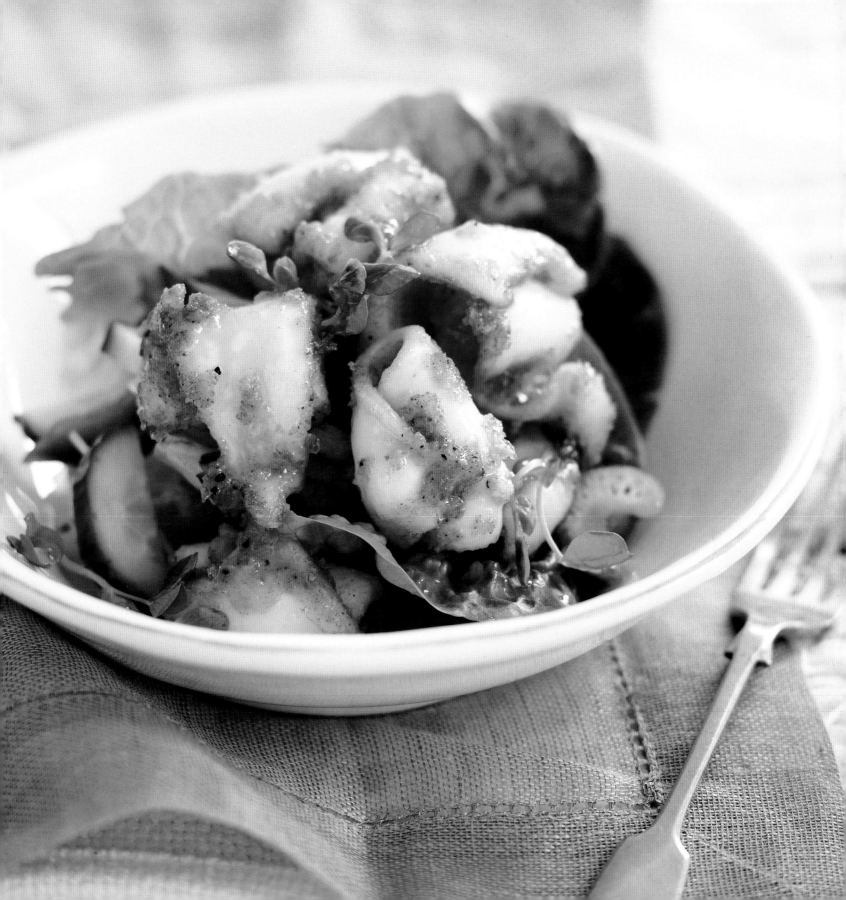

Lamb and sweet potato curry

SERVES 4

This lovely, rich dish achieves its depth of flavour without the use of onion, which is a standard ingredient in most curries. The lamb can be replaced with beef or veal if preferred, and pumpkin may be used in place of the sweet potato.

Combine the cornflour, paprika, garam masala, salt and pepper in a large bowl, add the lamb cubes and toss to coat.

Heat ⅓ cup (80 ml) oil in a large non-stick frying pan over medium heat, add the curry powder and heat for 1–2 minutes or until fragrant. Add the remaining oil, lamb pieces and celery to the pan and toss until browned on all sides. Stir in the tomato paste, stock and bay leaf. Increase the heat to high and bring to the boil, stirring well. Reduce the heat to medium–low, add the crushed tomatoes and simmer for 50–60 minutes or until the meat is tender.

Meanwhile, cook the sweet potato in a small saucepan of boiling water until just tender. Drain.

Add the sweet potato and spinach to the curry and stir until the spinach has wilted. Serve with steamed rice.

1 tablespoon maize cornflour

½ teaspoon paprika

½ teaspoon garam masala

salt and freshly ground black pepper

700 g lamb fillet, cut into 2.5 cm cubes

½ cup (125 ml) garlic-infused canola oil

1–2 tablespoons curry powder
   (gluten-free if on a gluten-free diet)

4 stalks celery, sliced

2 teaspoons tomato paste (puree)

2 cups (500 ml) onion-free beef stock
   (gluten-free if on a gluten-free diet)

1 bay leaf

1 × 425 g tin crushed tomatoes

2 sweet potatoes, cut into 1 cm cubes

2 cups (40 g) baby spinach leaves

steamed basmati rice, to serve

Beef korma

SERVES 4–6

There is nothing more rewarding than making a flavoursome dish from scratch, rather than relying on a prepared sauce. Try this sensational korma curry – you really will be able to tell the difference. If you have lactose intolerance, limit yourself to a half-serve only.

Heat the oil in a large heavy-based saucepan or stockpot over medium–high heat. Add the almonds, ginger and all the spices and stir for 30–60 seconds or until fragrant. Add the meat and toss to coat in the spices. Cook, stirring, for a few minutes or until browned on all sides.

Reduce the heat to low and cook for a further 5 minutes. Add half the yoghurt and sour cream, then cover and simmer gently for 2 hours or until the meat is tender, stirring regularly to prevent sticking. Stir in the remaining yoghurt and sour cream until heated through. Garnish with coriander and serve with rice.

⅓ cup (80 ml) garlic-infused canola oil

3 tablespoons ground almonds

2 teaspoons grated ginger

1½ teaspoon paprika

1 teaspoon ground coriander

1 teaspoon ground turmeric

½ teaspoon ground cinnamon

½ teaspoon ground cardamom

½ teaspoon chilli powder

½ teaspoon ground mace

¼ teaspoon ground cloves

1 kg beef fillet, cut into 2 cm cubes

1 cup (280 g) natural yoghurt

½ cup (120 g) sour cream

coriander leaves, to garnish

steamed rice, to serve

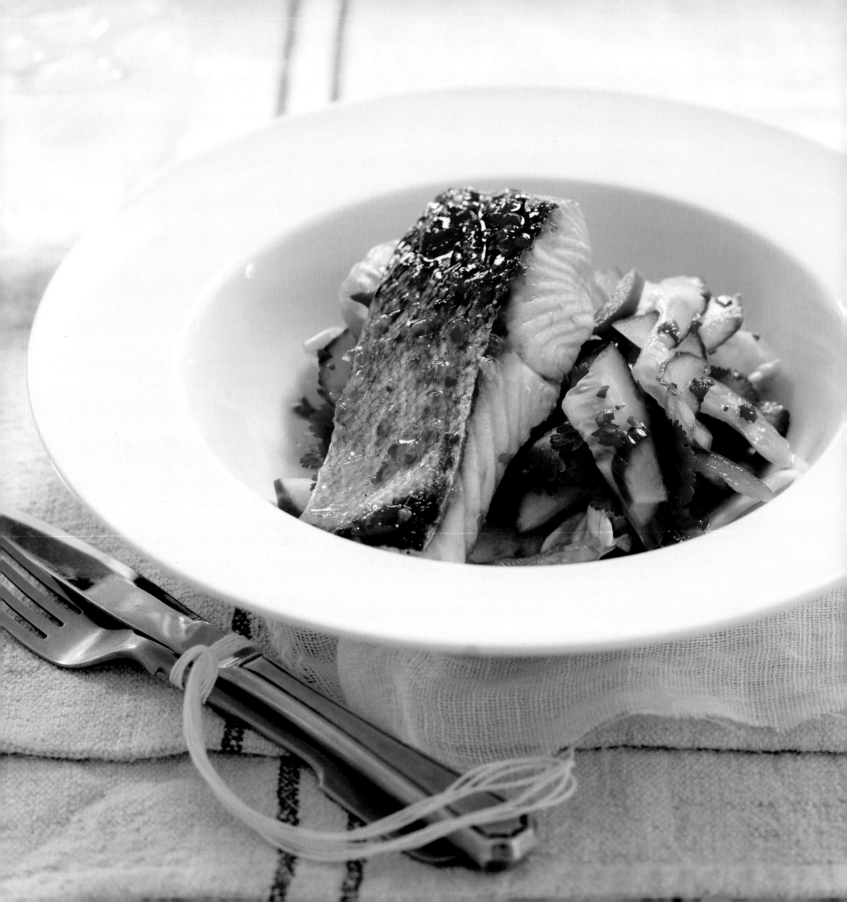

Chilli salmon with coriander salad

SERVES 4

Salmon is one of the richest sources of omega-3 fats, which are important for the prevention of heart disease. In particular, salmon contains a type of fat called DHA, which is important for brain development. The sweet chilli sauce is a simple flavour addition to this delicious and nutritious food from the sea.

Line a grill tray with foil. Place the salmon fillets on the tray, skin-side up, and cook under a hot grill for 1–2 minutes or until the skin becomes crispy. Reduce the heat to medium and turn the salmon over. Brush 1 teaspoon sweet chilli sauce over each piece of fish and season with salt and pepper. Grill for a further 3–4 minutes or until cooked to your liking.

Meanwhile, to make the salad, mix together the lettuce, cucumber, celery, capsicum and coriander in a large bowl. Combine the remaining ingredients in a small bowl and pour over the salad. Serve with the chilli salmon.

4 salmon fillets, skin on, pin bones removed
1 tablespoon sweet chilli sauce
salt and freshly ground black pepper

CORIANDER SALAD
150 g lettuce leaves, roughly chopped
½ large cucumber, halved lengthways and sliced
2 stalks celery, thinly sliced on the diagonal
½ green capsicum (pepper), thinly sliced
½ cup (25 g) firmly packed chopped coriander
½ small red chilli, finely chopped
2 tablespoons lime juice
1 tablespoon rice vinegar
2 tablespoons fish sauce
2 tablespoons brown sugar

Chicken kibbeh

SERVES 8–10

Kibbeh is a Middle Eastern dish made with cracked wheat (bulgur) and pine nuts. This recipes uses quinoa, a wheat-free alternative to bulgur with a similar texture. Unless you are feeding a crowd you will have leftovers, but don't worry – it freezes well!

Preheat the oven to 180°C. Grease and line a 25 cm × 30 cm baking tray.

Bring a medium saucepan of water to the boil and add the quinoa. Stir, then bring back to the boil and cook for 10–12 minutes or until just tender. Drain and rinse under cold water, then drain again.

To make the filling, combine all the ingredients in a small bowl.

Place the quinoa, chicken, oil, tarragon, allspice, tahini, salt and pepper in a bowl and mix until well combined. Divide into two portions. Press half the mixture into the base of the prepared baking tray and cover evenly with the filling. Top with the remaining kibbeh mixture, spreading it evenly over the filling.

Bake for 50–60 minutes or until cooked through – a skewer inserted into the centre should come out clean. Remove and rest for 5–10 minutes before cutting into squares. Garnish with the extra tarragon leaves and serve with salad.

1 cup (100 g) dried quinoa

1 kg minced chicken

2 tablespoons garlic-infused olive oil

3 tablespoons finely chopped tarragon, plus extra leaves to serve

2 teaspoons ground allspice

2 tablespoons tahini

salt and freshly ground black pepper

garden salad, to serve

FILLING

½ cup (80 g) pine nuts, toasted

3 small tomatoes, finely chopped

1 teaspoon ground cinnamon

1 cup (30 g) chopped flat-leaf parsley

1 teaspoon grated lemon zest

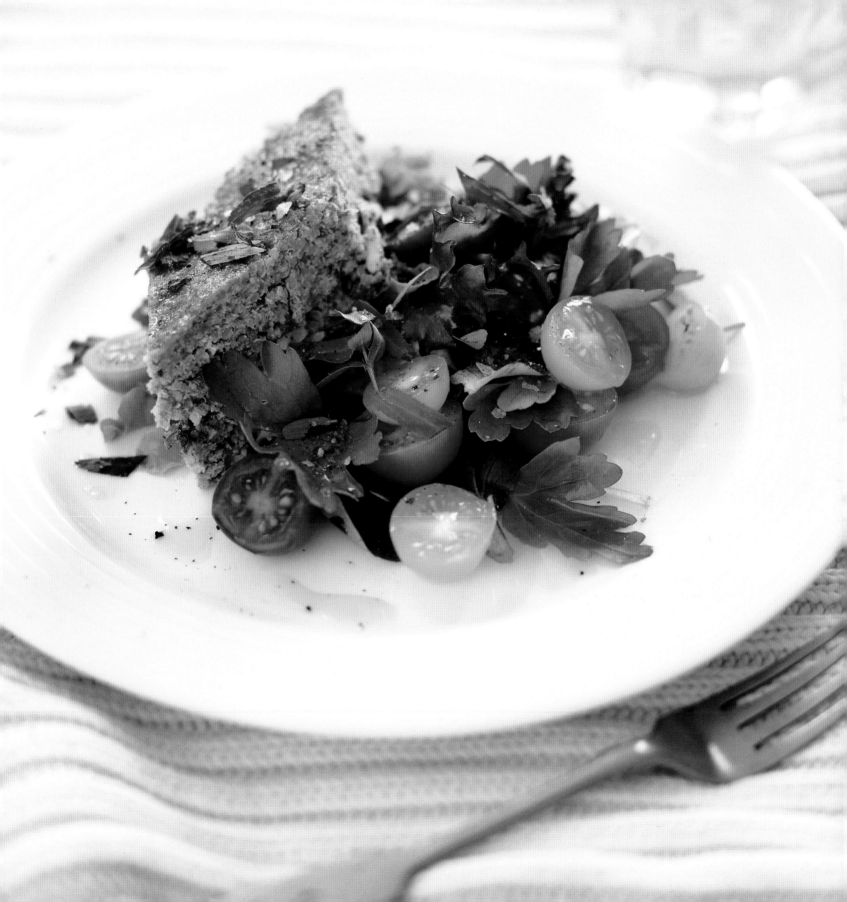

Singapore noodles

SERVES 4

If you have coeliac disease, use gluten-free curry powder, soy sauce and stock for this recipe. Those following the Low-FODMAP Diet who do not have coeliac disease don't have to take this precaution as the amount of wheat present should not cause any problems.

Soak the noodles in boiling water until soft. Rinse with cold water, then drain and set aside.

Heat the oils in a wok or frying pan over high heat until just smoking. Add the ginger and chilli and stir-fry for 30 seconds. Reduce the heat to medium–high, add the prawns and squid and stir-fry for 1 minute. Add the bean sprouts and pork and stir-fry for a further 2 minutes.

Make a well in the centre, pour in the beaten egg and cook, stirring to lightly scramble.

Add the remaining ingredients and the noodles and stir until all the liquid has been absorbed. Divide among four bowls, sprinkle with chives and serve.

1 cup (50 g) rice vermicelli noodles

2 tablespoons garlic-infused canola oil

2 tablespoons sesame oil

1 teaspoon grated ginger

1 small red chilli, finely chopped

100 g peeled raw prawns

5 small squid hoods, cleaned and thinly sliced

1 cup (80 g) bean sprouts

200 g pork fillet, thinly sliced

2 eggs, beaten

salt and freshly ground black pepper

3–4 teaspoons curry powder (gluten-free if on a gluten-free diet)

1 tablespoon soy sauce (gluten-free if on a gluten-free diet)

2 teaspoons brown sugar

3 tablespoons onion-free chicken stock (gluten-free if on a gluten-free diet)

chopped chives, to serve

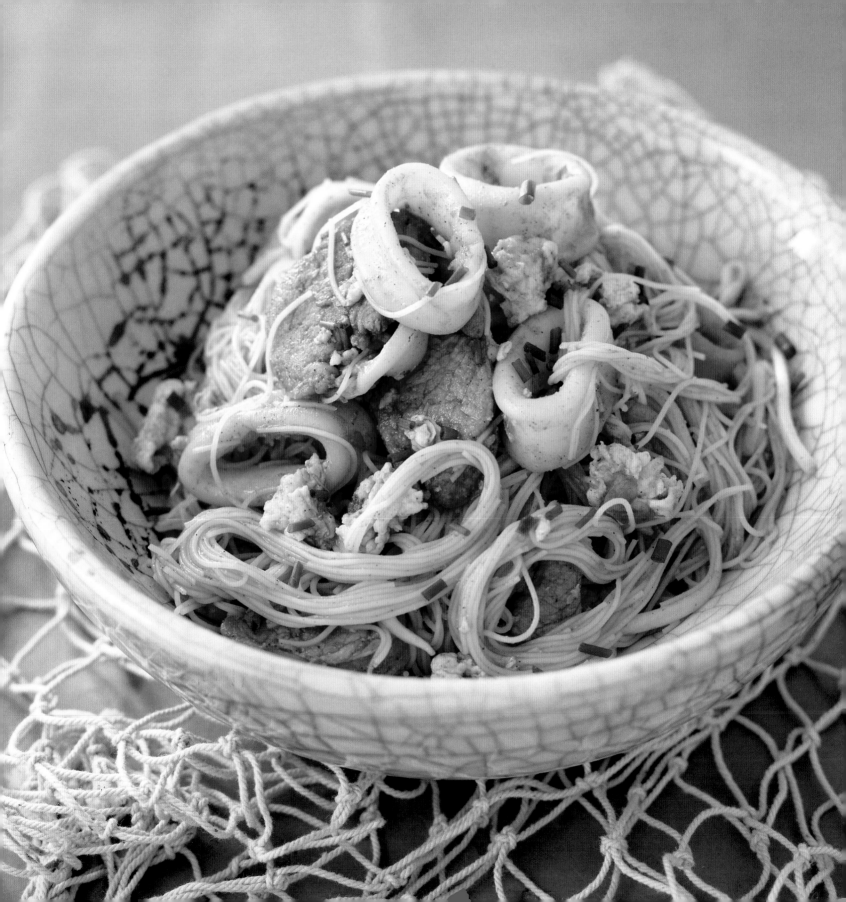

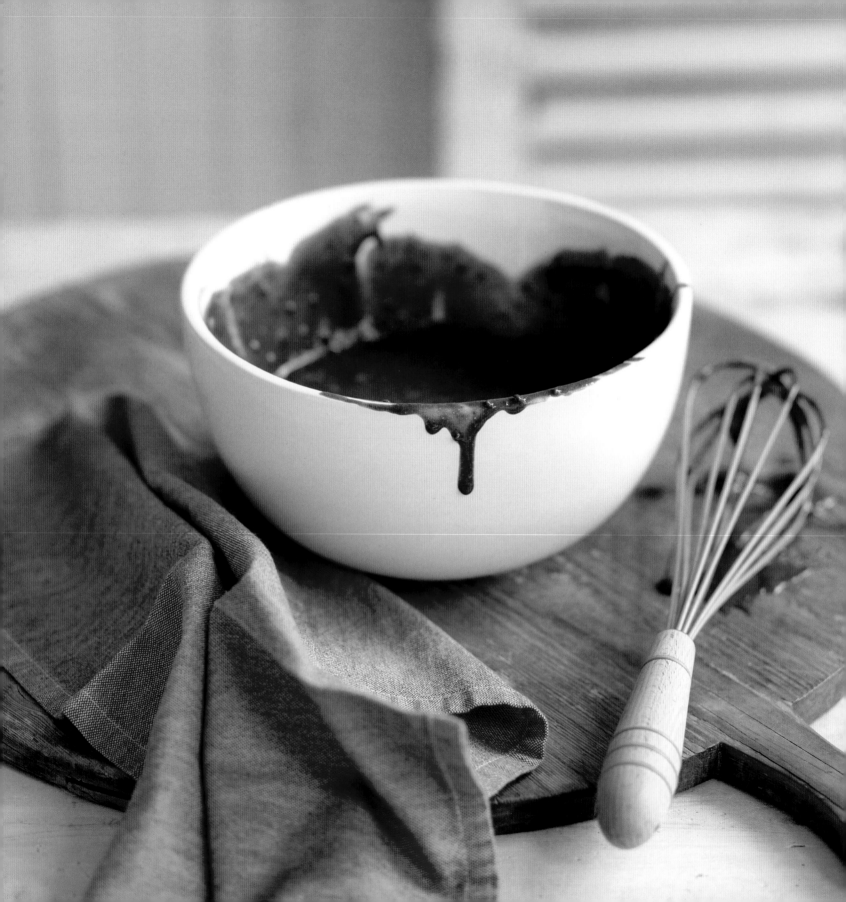

Baking

Poppy-seed, pepper and cheese sticks

MAKES ABOUT 30

For people with lactose intolerance, replace the cream cheese with soy cream cheese. The amount of soy flour used in this recipe is minimal so it will suit most people following the Low-FODMAP Diet. Assess your individual tolerance.

Place the cream cheese, butter and ½ cup (40 g) parmesan in a food processor and blend until smooth.

Sift the flours and xanthan gum three times into a large bowl (or mix well with a whisk to ensure they are well combined), then stir in the poppy seeds and pepper. Add the cream cheese mixture and mix with a metal spoon until just combined. Divide the dough into eight portions. Roll each portion on a flat surface to a 35 cm rope, then cut in half or into quarters.

Line a large baking tray with baking paper. Place the sticks on the tray and freeze for 20 minutes or until firm.

Preheat the oven to 180°C.

Bake the sticks for 12–15 minutes or until lightly golden brown and cooked through. Remove from the oven and allow to cool on the trays for 10 minutes before transferring to a clean tray. Spray with olive oil while still warm and roll in the remaining parmesan. Store in an airtight container for up to 7 days.

250 g cream cheese
80 g butter, softened
¾ cup (60 g) grated parmesan
½ cup (65 g) fine rice flour
3 tablespoons maize cornflour
3 tablespoons debittered soy flour
1 teaspoon xanthan gum
2 tablespoons poppy seeds
1 teaspoon coarsely ground
   black pepper

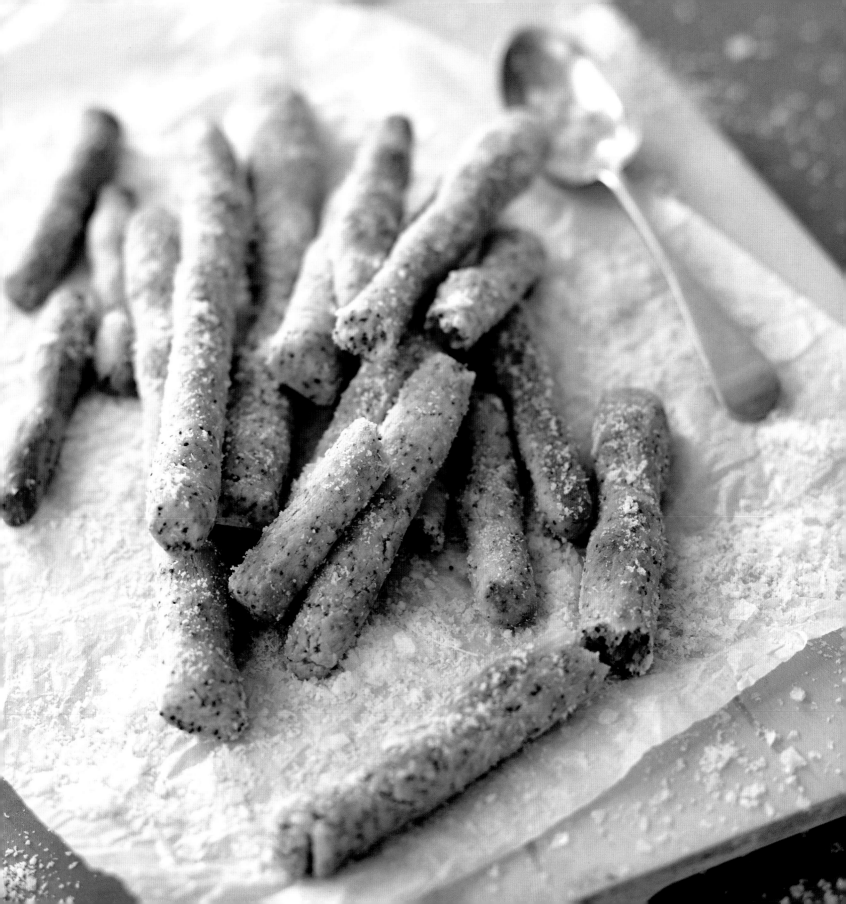

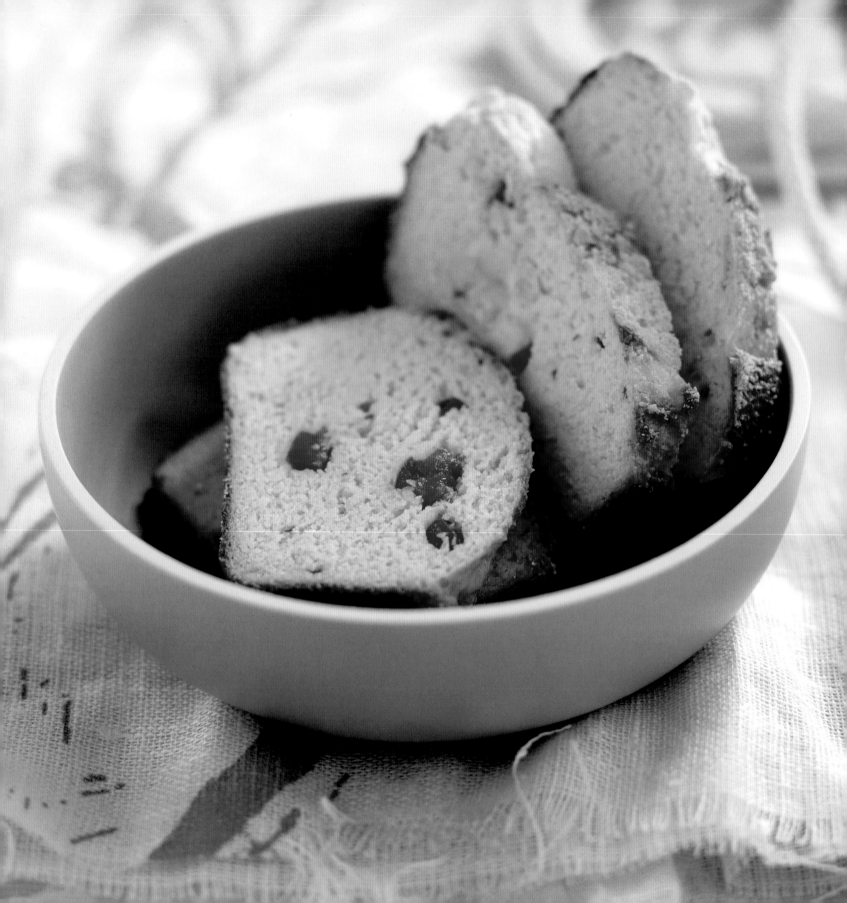

Chilli capsicum cornbread

SERVES 10

This savoury loaf is made with polenta, a coarse yellow meal made from corn that adds a grainy texture to baked foods. It is delicious served freshly baked from the oven, however any leftovers toast up superbly.

Preheat the oven to 180°C. Lightly grease a 20 cm × 9 cm loaf tin and line with baking paper.

Sift the flours, baking powder, bicarbonate of soda and xanthan gum three times into a bowl (or mix well with a whisk to ensure they are well combined). Stir in the polenta and salt.

Combine the egg, milk, oil, chilli, capsicum and three-quarters of the parmesan and add to the flour mixture. Mix well to combine, then pour into the loaf tin and sprinkle with the remaining cheese.

Bake for 35–45 minutes or until a skewer inserted into the centre comes out clean. Remove from the oven and allow to cool in the tin for 10 minutes before transferring to a wire rack to cool completely. Cut into slices and serve.

½ cup (65 g) fine rice flour
3 tablespoons maize cornflour
3 tablespoons potato flour
2 teaspoons baking powder
(gluten-free if on a gluten-free diet)
1 teaspoon bicarbonate of soda
1 teaspoon xanthan gum
1 cup (170 g) instant polenta
1 teaspoon salt
2 eggs, lightly beaten
1 cup (250 ml) milk
1 teaspoon olive oil
2 small red chillies, seeded and
finely chopped
½ red capsicum (pepper), seeded
and finely diced
1½ cups (120 g) grated parmesan

Zucchini and pepita cornmeal bread

SERVES 6

The grated zucchini keeps this loaf lovely and moist, while the pepitas give it a pleasing crunch. I like the parsley in the butter, but you can use other fresh herbs if preferred. The amount of soy flour used in this recipe is minimal so it will suit most people following the Low-FODMAP Diet. Assess your individual tolerance – if necessary, you can replace the soy flour with tapioca flour.

Preheat the oven to 200°C and line a baking tray with baking paper.

Sift the flours, baking powder, bicarbonate of soda and xanthan gum three times into a bowl (or mix well with a whisk to ensure they are well combined). Stir in the polenta, zucchini and pepitas. Make a well in the centre and add the warmed milk and melted butter. Season with salt and pepper and mix well with a wooden spoon.

Gently bring the dough together with your hands to form a soft ball. Turn out onto a clean surface dusted with gluten-free cornflour and knead until smooth.

Divide the dough in half, form into two balls and place on the baking tray. Brush with a little oil and sprinkle with sea salt, then bake for 20–25 minutes or until golden brown and cooked through.

To make the parsley butter, mix together the butter and parsley in a bowl. Serve with the warm bread.

1 cup (130 g) fine rice flour
¾ cup (135 g) potato flour
½ cup (45 g) debittered soy flour
2 teaspoons baking powder
   (gluten-free if on a gluten-free diet)
1 teaspoon bicarbonate of soda
1 teaspoon xanthan gum
1 cup (170 g) instant polenta
1 zucchini (courgette), grated and
   drained on paper towel
⅓ cup (65 g) pepitas
200 ml milk (rice, gluten-free soy
   or regular), warmed
40 g butter, melted
salt and freshly ground black pepper
olive oil, for brushing
sea salt flakes, for sprinkling

PARSLEY BUTTER

50 g butter
3 tablespoons chopped flat-leaf parsley

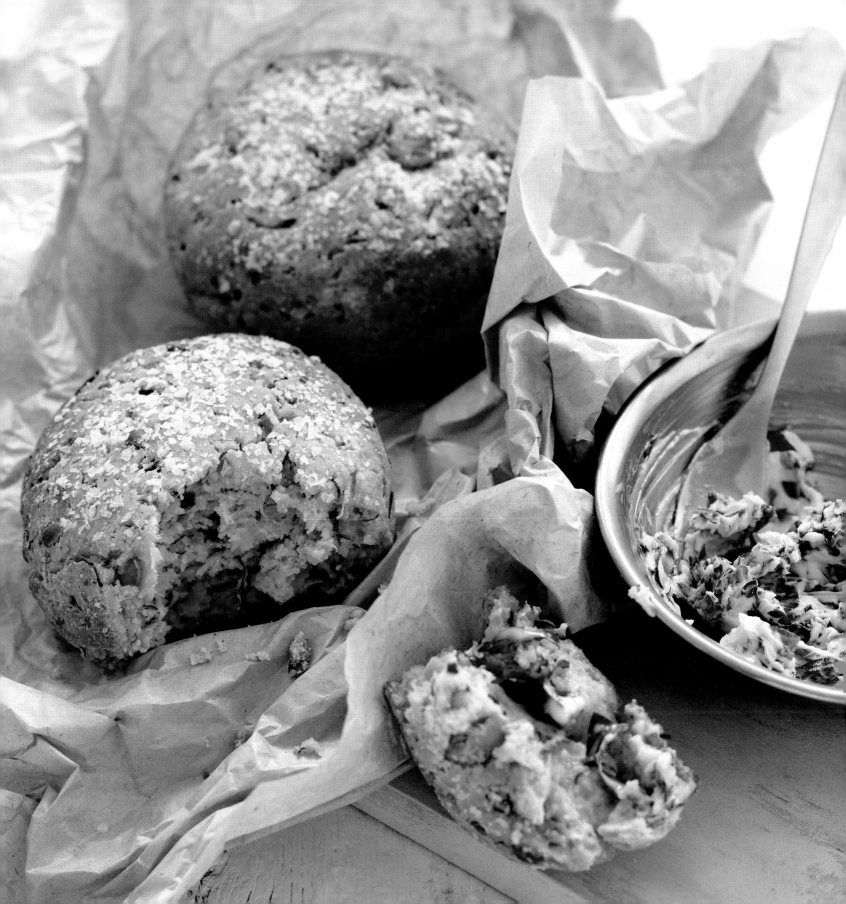

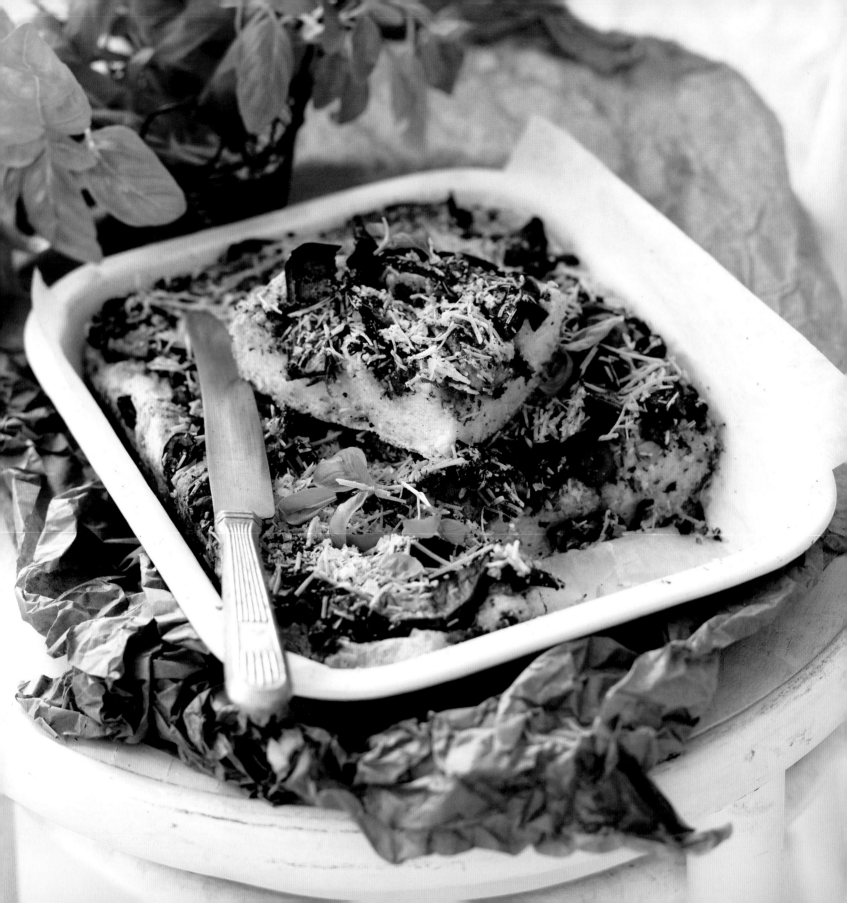

Olive and eggplant focaccia

SERVES 6–8

Things have come a long way in a few short years – these days, there is an abundance of gluten-free bread mixes available in supermarkets, health-food stores and other retail outlets. They all vary in taste and texture so you are sure to find one that suits you.

Preheat the oven to 180°C and line a deep baking tray with baking paper.

Make the gluten-free bread mix following the directions on the packet and spoon onto the tray. Using the back of a metal spoon, spread out the mixture to cover the tray (it should be about 2 cm thick).

Spread the pesto evenly over the bread mix (I usually do this with the back of a small metal spoon, dipping the spoon in water if required). Top with the olives, eggplant and parmesan, season with salt and pepper and bake for 25–35 minutes or until lightly browned. Remove from the oven and cool to room temperature in the tray. Cut into pieces and serve warm, sprinkled with the basil leaves.

1 cup (280 g) gluten-free bread mix
3 tablespoons basil pesto (gluten-free if on a gluten-free diet)
½ cup (75 g) sliced kalamata olives
100 g marinated grilled eggplant (aubergine) slices, roughly chopped
½ cup (40 g) grated parmesan
salt and freshly ground black pepper
small basil leaves, to garnish

Choc chip biscuits

MAKES 18

The amount of soy flour used here is minimal so these biscuits should suit most people following the Low-FODMAP Diet. Assess your individual tolerance.

Preheat the oven to 180°C and line two baking trays with baking paper.

Beat the butter and brown sugar with electric beaters until creamy. Add the eggs one at a time, beating well between additions.

Sift the flours and xanthan gum three times into a bowl (or mix well with a whisk to ensure they are well combined). Add to the butter mixture and stir until well combined. Mix in the choc chips, then gently bring the dough together with your hands. Roll into golf-ball-sized balls and place on the trays, about 5 cm apart (to allow for spreading). Flatten slightly with the back of a fork.

Bake for 12–15 minutes or until golden. Cool on the trays for 10 minutes before transferring to a wire rack to cool completely.

200 g unsalted butter, softened
¾ cup (165 g) brown sugar
2 eggs
1¼ cups (160 g) fine rice flour
⅓ cup (50 g) maize cornflour
½ cup (45 g) debittered soy flour
1 teaspoon xanthan gum
150 g choc chips (white, milk or dark, or use a mixture)

Macaroons

MAKES 40

Macaroons are a flourless biscuit that can be adapted to suit your tastes by, for example, adding desiccated coconut or cocoa. They keep very well in an airtight container for up to a week.

Preheat the oven to 140°C and line two baking trays with baking paper.

Combine the ground almonds and baking powder in a small bowl.

In a separate bowl, beat the egg white with electric beaters until firm. Gradually beat in the sugar, then continue beating for 5 minutes or until stiff peaks form. Add the ground almond mix, almond essence and melted butter and mix with a metal spoon.

Roll 2 teaspoons of dough per biscuit into a ball. Place on the trays, allowing room for spreading, and flatten slightly. Bake for 25 minutes. Cool on the trays for 5 minutes before transferring to a wire rack to cool completely.

¾ cup (90 g) ground almonds
½ teaspoon gluten-free baking powder
1 egg white
½ cup (110 g) caster sugar
3 drops of almond essence
20 g unsalted butter, melted

Choc chip biscuits →

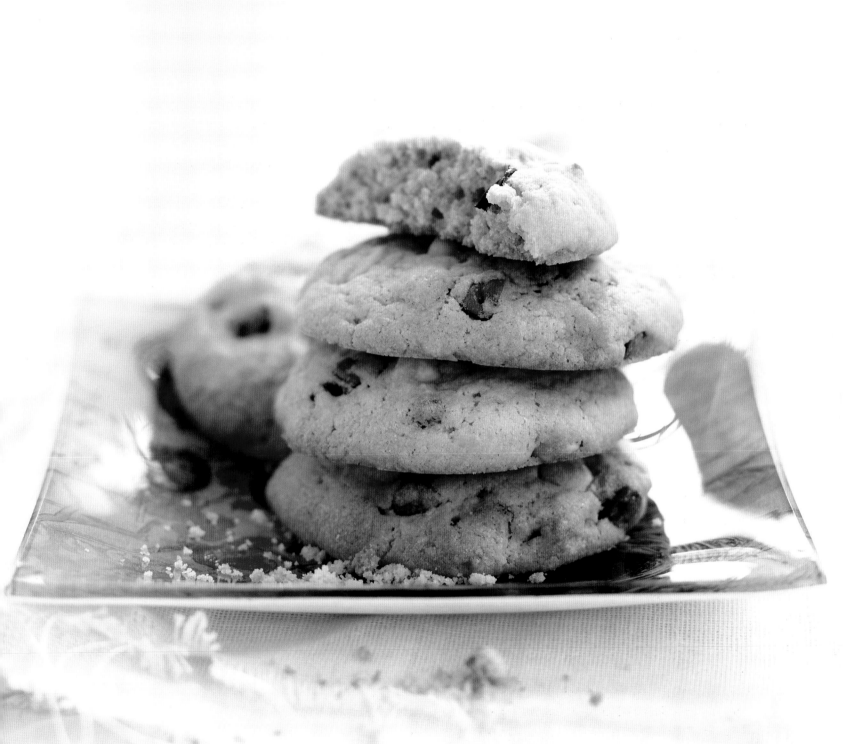

Sultana scones

MAKES 14

At last there is a way for people following the Low-FODMAP Diet to
tenjoy this much-loved afternoon-tea favourite. And if you prefer your
scones plain, simply omit the sultanas. The amount of soy flour used
in this recipe is minimal so it will suit most people following the
Low-FODMAP Diet. Assess your individual tolerance.

Preheat the oven to 200°C. Grease a baking tray and dust with gluten-free
cornflour.

Sift the flours, xanthan gum, baking powder and sugar three times into a
large bowl (or mix well with a whisk to ensure they are well combined). Rub in
the butter with your fingertips until the mixture resembles fine breadcrumbs.
Add the sultanas and mix to combine.

Whisk the milk and egg in a bowl. Add to the sultana mixture and mix with
a metal spoon until the dough begins to hold together. Gently bring the dough
together with your hands and turn out onto a lightly floured surface. Knead
gently four or five times with your hands (by pressing and then turning) until
the dough is just smooth.

Roll out the dough to a thickness of about 3 cm. Using a 5 cm fluted or
plain cutter, cut out the scones. Make sure you use a straight-down motion
to do this – if you twist the cutter the scones will rise unevenly during cooking.
It also helps to dip the cutter in cornflour before each cut.

Place the scones on the baking tray about 1 cm apart. Brush the tops with
a little extra milk and bake for 15–18 minutes or until golden and cooked
through. Turn the tray around halfway through baking. Remove the scones
from the oven and immediately wrap them in a clean tea towel (this will help
give them a soft crust). Serve warm with jam and whipped cream.

2 cups (300 g) maize cornflour
2 cups (250 g) tapioca flour
1 cup (90 g) debittered soy flour
2 teaspoons xanthan gum
1 tablespoon baking powder
    (gluten-free if on a gluten-free diet)
½ cup (110 g) caster sugar
150 g unsalted butter, at room
    temperature, cut into cubes
3 tablespoons sultanas
300 ml low-fat milk
2 eggs
2 tablespoons milk, extra
jam and whipped cream, to serve

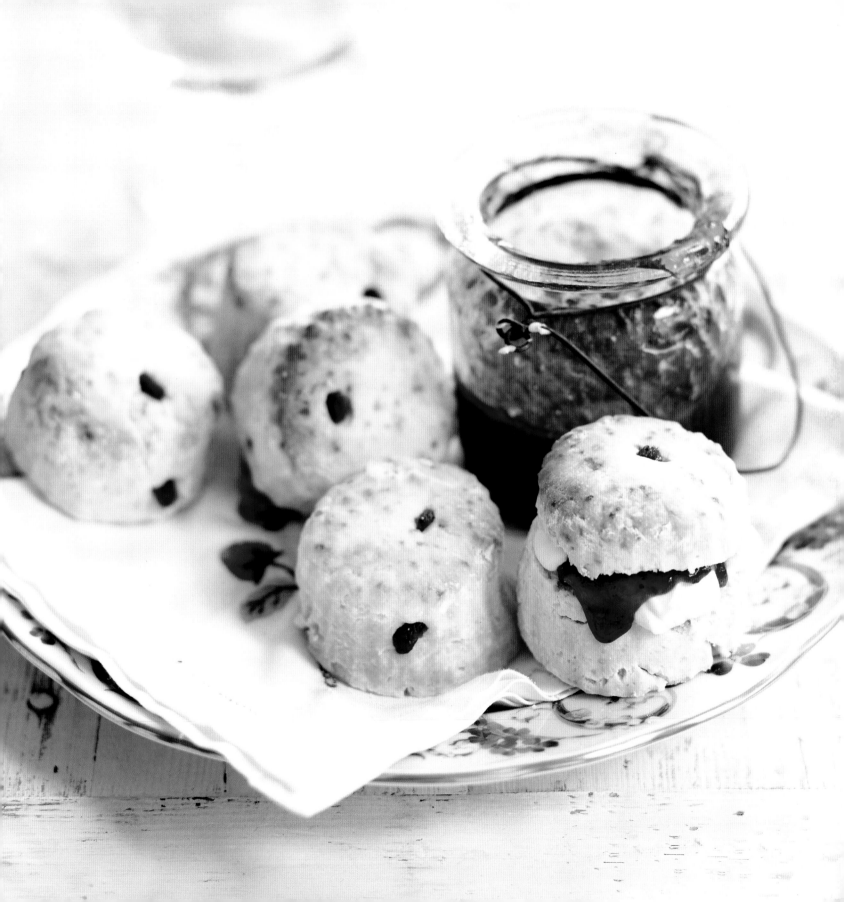

Simple sweet biscuits

MAKES 20

These versatile biscuits are delicious on their own, or can be crushed to make biscuit bases for cheesecakes and slices. See, for example, Strawberry slice on page 230, New York cheesecake on page 236 and Baked caramel cheesecake on page 220. The amount of soy flour used in this recipe is minimal so it will suit most people following the Low-FODMAP Diet. Assess your individual tolerance.

Preheat the oven to 170°C and grease two baking trays.

Place the butter and sugars in a bowl and cream with electric beaters. Add the egg and vanilla and beat well.

Sift the flours and bicarbonate of soda three times into a bowl (or mix well with a whisk to ensure they are well combined). Add to the butter mixture and beat well.

Place tablespoonfuls of mixture on the trays, allowing room for spreading, and bake for 8–10 minutes or until golden brown. Remove from the oven and leave to cool on the trays for 5 minutes before transferring to a wire rack to cool completely.

125 g unsalted butter

3 tablespoons brown sugar

3 tablespoons caster sugar

1 egg

1 teaspoon vanilla essence

⅔ cup (85 g) fine rice flour

½ cup (75 g) maize cornflour

3 tablespoons debittered soy flour

½ teaspoon bicarbonate of soda

Basic chocolate cake

SERVES 10–12

This is a family chocolate cake that everyone will enjoy – I know this from experience! People following a lactose-free diet should choose lactose-free milk and yoghurt.

Preheat the oven to 170°C and grease a 23 cm springform tin.

Sift the flours, cocoa powder, baking powder, bicarbonate of soda and xanthan gum three times into a large bowl (or mix well with a whisk to ensure they are well combined).

Whisk the eggs and sugar until thick and foamy. Add the melted butter, yoghurt and milk and stir until well combined. Pour this mixture into the sifted flours and beat with electric beaters for 2–3 minutes.

Pour the batter into the tin and bake for 45–55 minutes or until firm to touch (a skewer inserted into the centre should come out clean). Cover with foil halfway through to prevent overbrowning. Remove from the oven and allow to cool in the tin for 5 minutes before transferring to a wire rack to cool completely.

Dust with icing sugar and serve with a dollop of cream.

170 g fine rice flour

½ cup (75 g) maize cornflour

½ cup (90 g) potato flour

⅔ cup (70 g) cocoa powder

2 teaspoons baking powder
(gluten-free if on a gluten-free diet)

1 teaspoon bicarbonate of soda

1 teaspoon xanthan gum

2 eggs

1½ cups (330 g) sugar

50 g unsalted butter, melted

200 g vanilla yoghurt (gluten-free
if on a gluten-free diet)

⅔ cup (170 ml) low-fat milk

pure icing sugar, for dusting

thick cream, to serve

Mocha mud cake

SERVES 12–14

The secret of this delicious chocolate cake is the subtle coffee flavour in the background. Those who love a stronger coffee hit may wish to increase the quantity to enhance the impact of this feature ingredient. There are no raising agents in this recipe – it will remain a low non-rising cake, the way a good mud cake should be! Rich and dense, a small serve is all that is needed.

Preheat the oven to 160°C. Grease and line a 20 cm round cake tin.

Place the coffee, chocolate, butter, vanilla and cocoa powder in a medium glass bowl. Set over a saucepan of simmering water (make sure the base of the bowl does not touch the water) and stir until melted and well combined.

Place the sugar and eggs in a large bowl and beat with electric beaters on high for 3–5 minutes or until light, fluffy and doubled in volume. Gradually fold in the chocolate mixture, stirring gently with a metal spoon to combine.

Sift the flours and xanthan gum three times into a large bowl (or mix well with a whisk to ensure they are well combined). Gradually fold into the chocolate mixture with a metal spoon.

Pour the batter into the tin and bake for 50–60 minutes or until a skewer inserted into the centre comes out clean. Remove from the oven and allow to cool in the tin for 15 minutes before transferring to a wire rack to cool completely. Dust with extra cocoa powder if liked and serve.

3 tablespoons strong coffee

200 g dark chocolate bits

180 g butter, chopped

1 teaspoon vanilla extract

⅓ cup (35 g) cocoa powder, plus extra for dusting (optional)

1 cup (220 g) caster sugar

3 eggs

½ cup (65 g) fine rice flour

¼ cup (45 g) potato flour

¼ cup (40 g) maize cornflour

1 teaspoon xanthan gum

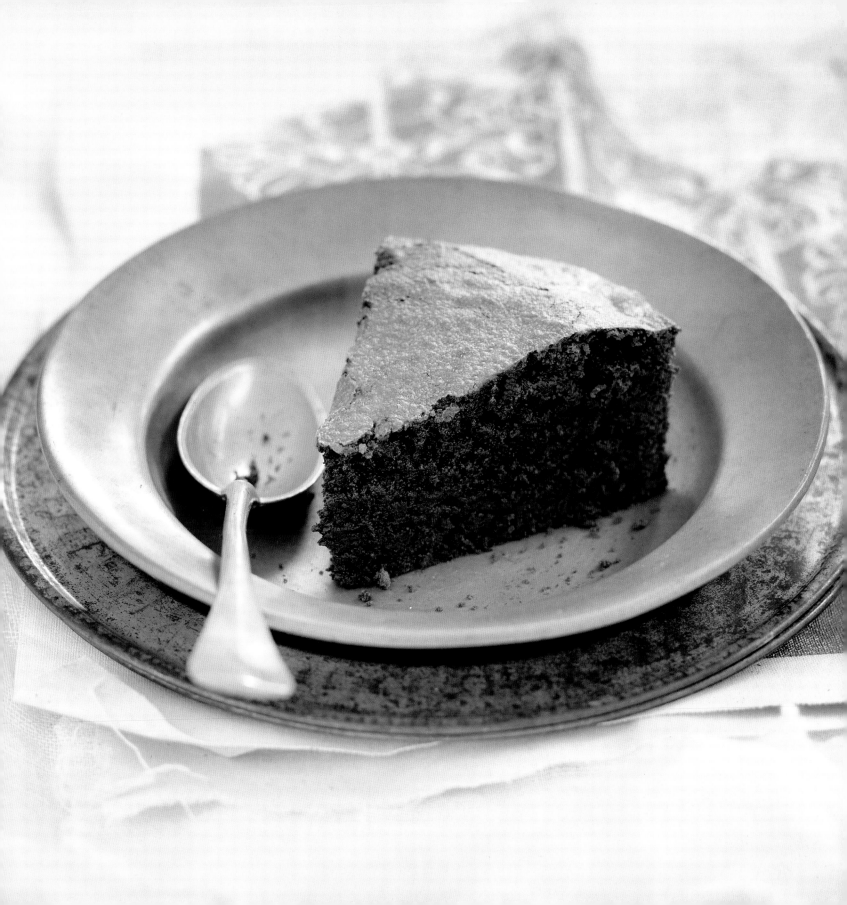

Vanilla cake

SERVES 10–12

It is preferable to use fine rice flour for baking, as regular rice flour can give quite a grainy mouth-feel. Fine rice flour is available from Asian grocers and many larger supermarkets. For people with lactose intolerance, make sure you use lactose-free yoghurt and milk.

Preheat the oven to 170°C and grease a 23 cm springform tin.

Sift the flours, baking powder, bicarbonate of soda and xanthan gum three times into a large bowl (or mix well with a whisk to ensure they are well combined).

Whisk together the eggs, sugar and vanilla until thick and foamy. Add the melted butter, yoghurt and milk and stir until well combined. Pour into the sifted flours and beat with electric beaters for 2–3 minutes.

Pour the batter into the tin and bake for 30–35 minutes or until firm to touch (a skewer inserted into the centre should come out clean). Remove from the oven and allow to cool in the tin for 5 minutes before transferring to a wire rack to cool completely. Dust with icing sugar and serve.

1 cup (130 g) fine rice flour
½ cup (75 g) gluten-free custard powder
½ cup (90 g) potato flour
2 teaspoons baking powder (gluten-free if on a gluten-free diet)
1 teaspoon bicarbonate of soda
1 teaspoon xanthan gum
2 eggs
1 cup (220 g) sugar
3 teaspoons vanilla essence
50 g butter, melted
200 g vanilla yoghurt (gluten-free if on a gluten-free diet)
⅔ cup (170 ml) low-fat milk
pure icing sugar, for dusting

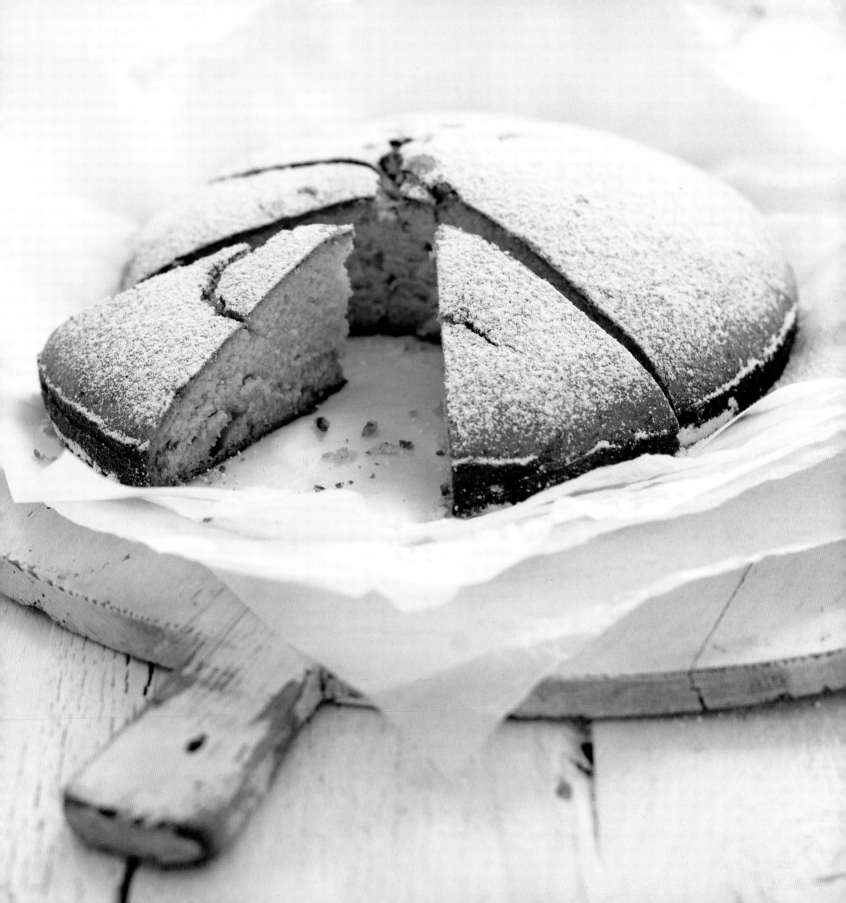

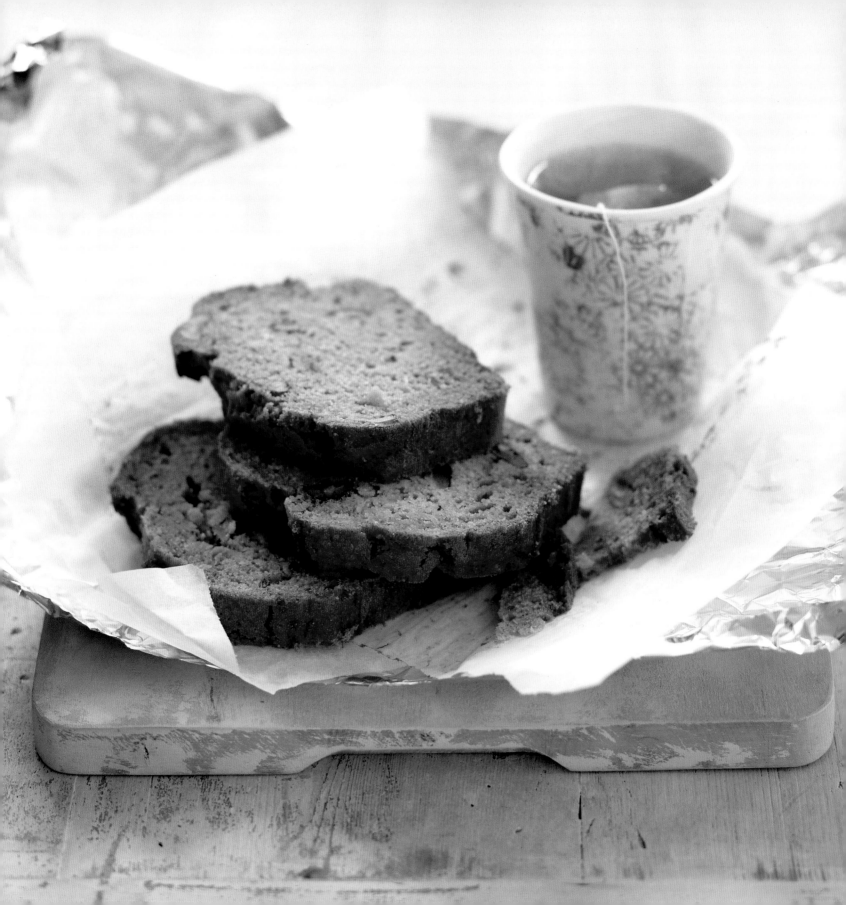

Carrot and pecan cake

SERVES 10

This moist, flavoursome cake needs no adornment and is perfect to enjoy for morning or afternoon tea. Tapioca flour can be purchased at Asian grocers and in the Asian section of larger supermarkets. You may wish to add chopped glace ginger pieces, a small handful of dried cranberries or sultanas, or 2 tablespoons mixed spice as variations to this great flavour base.

Preheat the oven to 170°C. Grease and line a 20 cm × 9 cm loaf tin.

Sift together the flours, cinnamon, bicarbonate of soda, baking powder and xanthan gum three times into a medium bowl (or mix well with a whisk to ensure they are well combined). Stir in the brown sugar and chopped pecans. Add the grated carrot, oil, egg and milk and mix well with a wooden spoon.

Spoon the batter into the tin and smooth the surface. Bake for about 1 hour or until golden brown (a skewer inserted into the centre should come out clean). Cover with foil halfway through to prevent overbrowning. Remove from the oven and leave to cool in the tin for 10 minutes before transferring to a wire rack to cool completely.

1 cup (130 g) fine rice flour
½ cup (75 g) maize cornflour
½ cup (65 g) tapioca flour
2 teaspoons ground cinnamon
1 teaspoon bicarbonate of soda
2 teaspoons baking powder
(gluten-free if on a gluten-free diet)
1 teaspoon xanthan gum
1 cup (220 g) brown sugar
¾ cup (90 g) chopped pecan pieces
2 small carrots, grated
½ cup (125 ml) vegetable oil
3 eggs, lightly beaten
½ cup (125 ml) low-fat milk

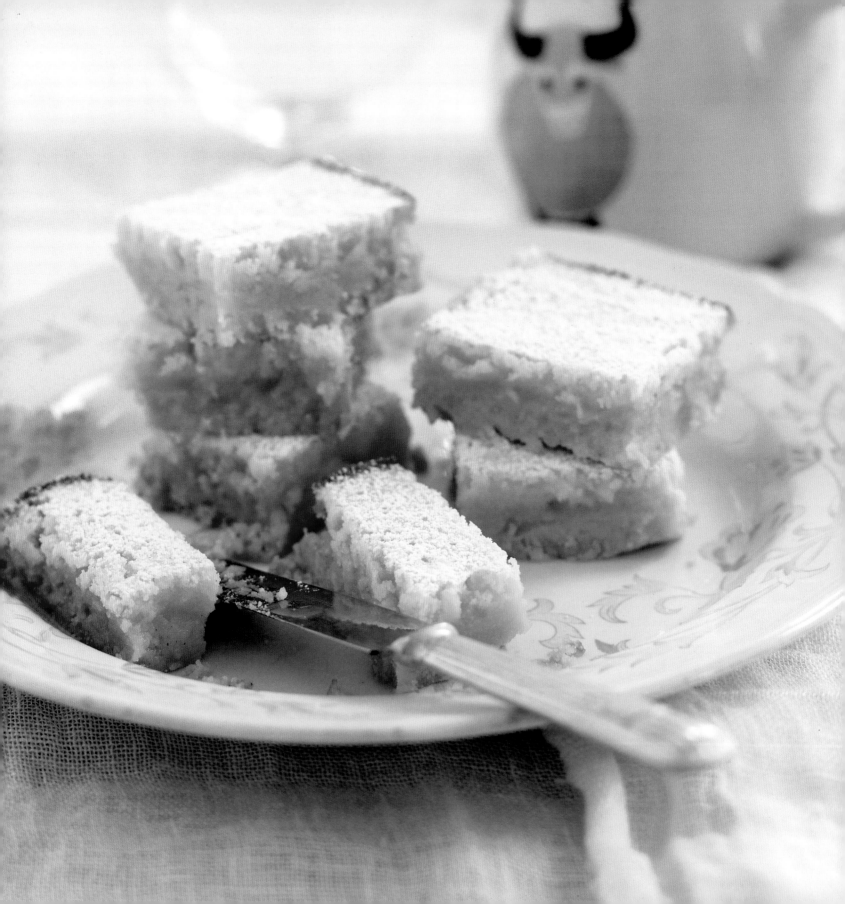

Lemon lime slice

MAKES 20 PIECES

This one is for those who love a sweet treat with a zesty twist. You'll want to start eating it as soon as it is baked, but try to resist the temptation – it behaves a lot better if you let it cool before slicing. The amount of soy flour used in this recipe is minimal so it will suit most people following the Low-FODMAP Diet. Assess your individual tolerance.

Preheat the oven to 160°C. Grease and line an 18 cm square cake tin with baking paper.

Place the flours, sugar and lemon zest in a food processor and process until just combined. Add the butter, one piece at a time, until the mixture comes together in a ball. Remove and press into the tin. Bake for 10 minutes or until lightly browned. Reduce the oven temperature to 150°C.

To make the topping, beat the eggs and sugar with electric beaters until well combined but not thickened. Add the lemon and lime juice, lemon zest and flour and mix with a metal spoon.

Pour the topping over the base and bake for 25–30 minutes or until golden. Allow to cool in the tin before cutting into slices. Dust with icing sugar just before serving.

¾ cup (100 g) fine rice flour
½ cup (45 g) debittered soy flour
½ cup (110 g) caster sugar
2 teaspoons grated lemon zest
125 g unsalted butter, chilled, roughly chopped
pure icing sugar, for dusting

TOPPING
3 eggs
¾ cup (165 g) caster sugar
3 tablespoons lemon juice
3 tablespoons lime juice
1 teaspoon grated lemon zest
3 tablespoons fine rice flour

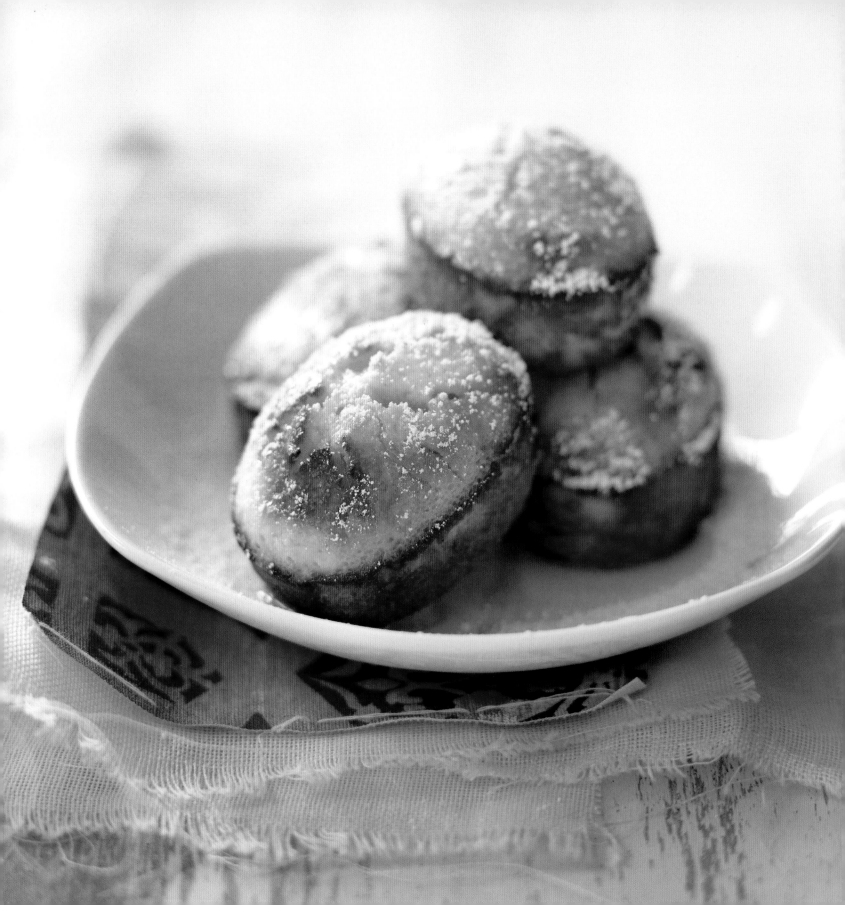

Lemon friands

MAKES 12

These miniature almond cakes are a delight on their own or simply dusted with icing sugar. If you want to dress them up, the lemon glaze makes a delicious addition.

Preheat the oven to 180°C. Lightly grease 12 friand tins (or petite loaf tins).

Melt the butter in a small saucepan over low heat, then cook for 3–4 minutes until you start to see flecks of brown appear. Remove from the heat.

Sift the icing sugar and flours three times into a bowl (or mix well with a whisk to ensure they are well combined) and stir in the ground almonds and lemon zest. Add the egg whites, lemon juice, vanilla and melted butter and mix well with a metal spoon.

Spoon the mixture into the tins to two-thirds full. Bake for 12–15 minutes until light golden and firm to touch. Remove from the oven and leave to cool in the tins for 5 minutes before transferring to a wire rack to cool completely.

Meanwhile, to make the glaze, place all the ingredients and 2 tablespoons hot water in a small heavy-based saucepan over low heat and cook, stirring constantly, for 10 minutes or until thickened. Remove from the heat and cool to room temperature.

Drizzle the lemon glaze over the friands and dust with icing sugar.

140 g unsalted butter
2 cups (320 g) pure icing sugar, plus extra for dusting
3 tablespoons maize cornflour
3 tablespoons rice flour
1¼ cups (150 g) ground almonds
finely grated zest of 1 lemon
5 egg whites, lightly whisked
2 tablespoons lemon juice
1 teaspoon vanilla essence

LEMON GLAZE
juice of 1 lemon
1 teaspoon finely grated lemon zest
⅓ cup (75 g) caster sugar
40 g unsalted butter
½ teaspoon gluten-free cornflour

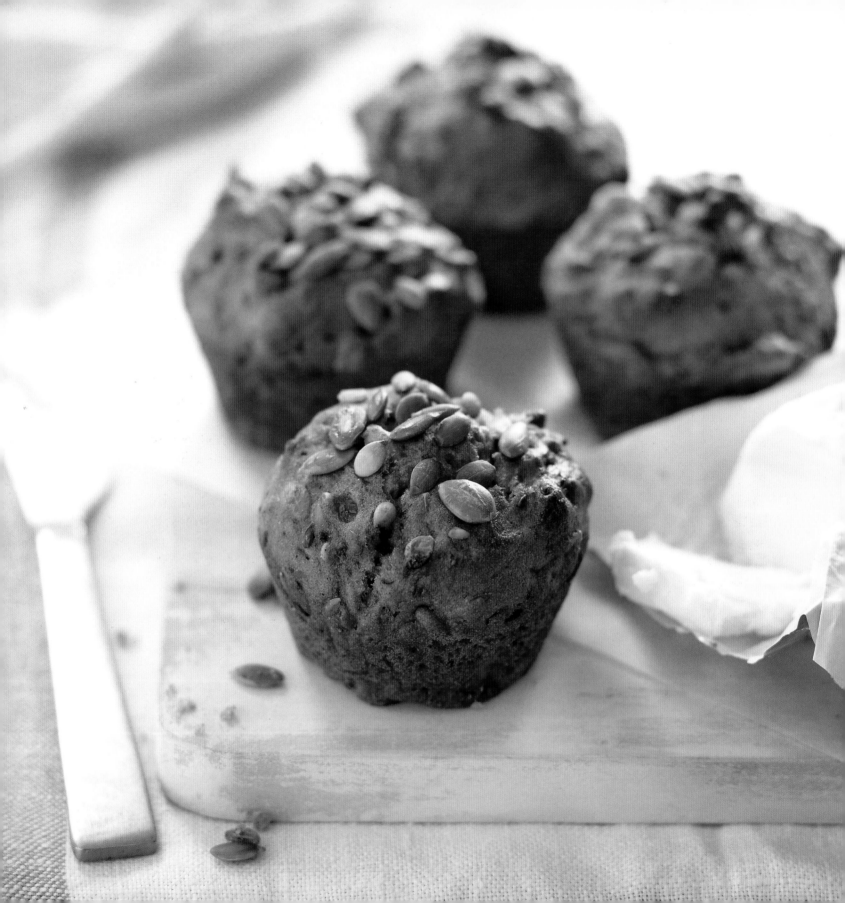

Chia seed and spice muffins

MAKES 12

Chia seeds are packed with nutrition, making them a wholesome snack, full of goodness and crunch. You could also spoon the mixture into eight Texas muffin tins and enjoy these fragrant muffins for lunch. The amount of soy flour in this recipe is minimal so it will suit most people following the Low-FODMAP Diet. Assess your individual tolerance – if necessary, replace the soy flour with tapioca flour.

Preheat the oven to 170°C. Grease a 12-hole standard muffin tin.

Sift the flours, baking powder, bicarbonate of soda, mixed spice, cinnamon and xanthan gum three times into a large bowl (or mix well with a whisk to ensure they are well combined).

Place the eggs, oil, milk, chia seeds, sunflower kernels, pepitas and brown sugar in a medium bowl and mix with a wooden spoon until well combined. Pour into the sifted flours and mix well with a wooden spoon for 2–3 minutes.

Spoon the mixture into the muffin holes to two-thirds full and sprinkle the extra pepitas evenly over the top. Bake for 20–25 minutes or until firm to touch (a skewer inserted into the centre should come out clean). Remove from the oven and allow to cool in the tin for 5 minutes before transferring to a wire rack to cool completely.

1 cup (140 g) brown rice flour
½ cup (75 g) maize cornflour
½ cup (45 g) debittered soy flour
2 teaspoons baking powder
   (gluten-free if on a gluten-free diet)
1 teaspoon bicarbonate of soda
2 tablespoons mixed spice
1 tablespoon ground cinnamon
1 teaspoon xanthan gum
3 eggs
½ cup (125 ml) vegetable oil
½ cup (125 ml) low-fat milk
⅓ cup (40 g) chia seeds
½ cup (80 g) sunflower kernels
½ cup (100 g) pepitas
½ cup (110 g) brown sugar
2 tablespoons pepitas, extra

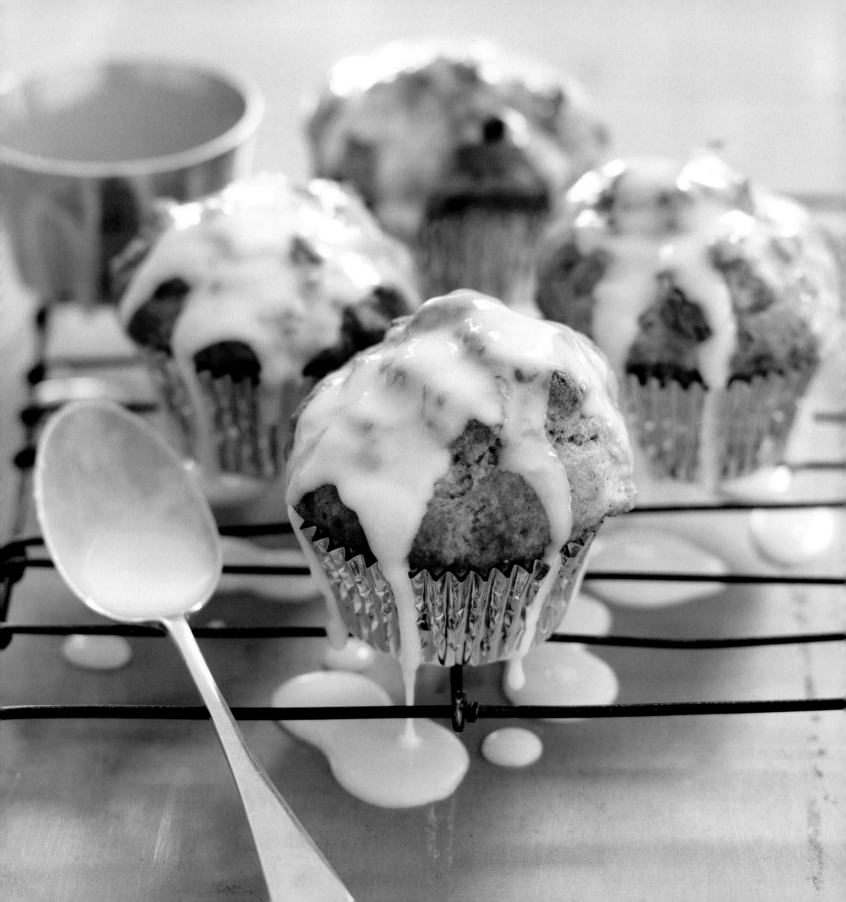

Pineapple muffins

MAKES 12

The crushed pineapple through these muffins adds a sweet flavour and moist texture that's hard to resist. Any muffins that don't disappear immediately can be frozen for another time.

Preheat the oven to 180°C. Line a 12-hole standard muffin tin with patty cases.

Sift the flours, bicarbonate of soda, baking powder and xanthan gum three times into a medium bowl (or mix well with a whisk to ensure they are well combined). Add the sultanas and sugar.

Place the eggs in a bowl and beat with a metal spoon. Stir in the melted butter, pineapple and yoghurt, then fold into the flour mixture.

Spoon the batter into the patty cases and bake for 15–20 minutes, or until a skewer inserted into the centre of the muffins comes out clean. Remove from the oven and leave to cool in the tin for 5 minutes before transferring to a wire rack to cool completely.

Combine the icing sugar with enough of the reserved pineapple liquid to form a smooth, spreadable icing. Drizzle over the cooled muffins and serve.

1 cup (130 g) fine rice flour

½ cup (75 g) maize cornflour

½ cup (90 g) potato flour

1 teaspoon bicarbonate of soda

2 teaspoons baking powder
(gluten-free if on a gluten-free diet)

1 teaspoon xanthan gum

3 tablespoons sultanas

½ cup (110 g) caster sugar

2 eggs

80 g unsalted butter, melted

440 g tinned crushed pineapple,
drained (reserve the liquid)

200 g vanilla yoghurt (gluten-free
if on a gluten-free diet)

1 cup (160 g) pure icing sugar, sifted

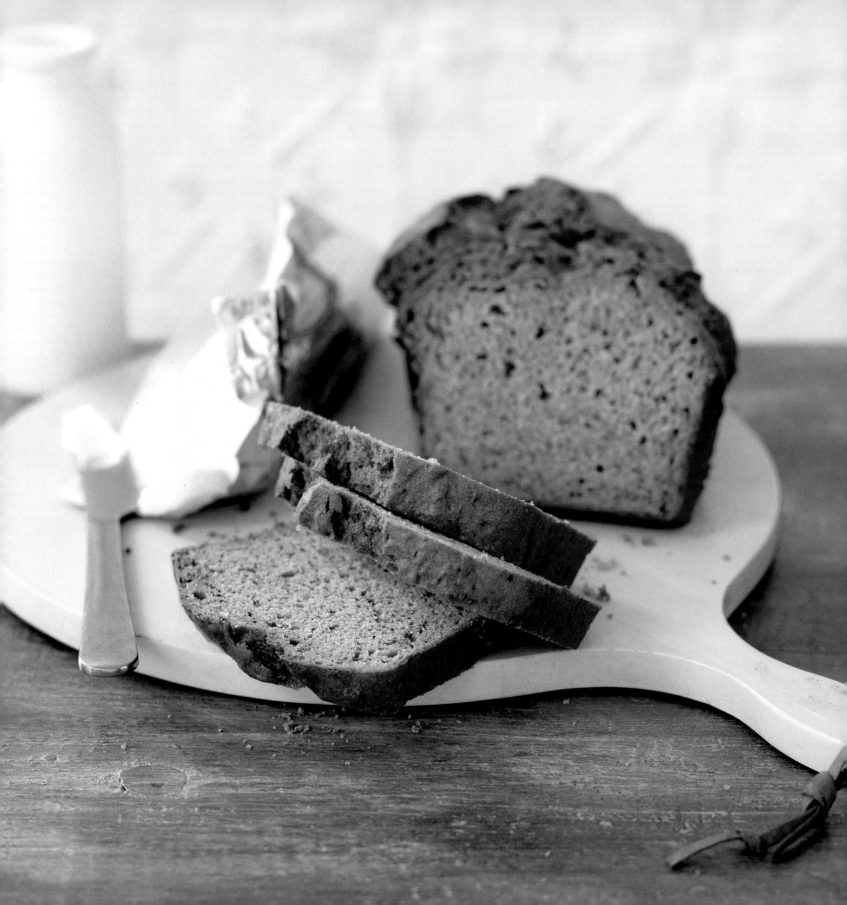

Moist banana cake

SERVES 12

This fragrant cake is delicious served warm. For an extra treat, spread it with a little butter which will melt beautifully into the moist cake.

Preheat the oven to 170°C and grease a 20 cm × 9 cm loaf tin.

Sift the flours, bicarbonate of soda, baking powder, xanthan gum and spices three times into a large bowl (or mix well with a whisk to ensure they are well combined).

Mix together the oil, yoghurt and eggs in a medium bowl, then stir in the mashed banana and brown sugar. Add to the dry ingredients and beat with electric beaters for 2–3 minutes.

Pour the batter into the tin and bake for 45–55 minutes or until golden brown (a skewer inserted into the centre should come out clean). Cover with foil halfway through to prevent overbrowning. Remove from the oven and leave to cool in the tin for 5 minutes before transferring to a wire rack to cool completely. Serve as is or spread with butter.

1 cup (130 g) fine rice flour

½ cup (75 g) maize cornflour

½ cup (90 g) potato flour

1 teaspoon bicarbonate of soda

2 teaspoons baking powder (gluten-free if on a gluten-free diet)

1 teaspoon xanthan gum

2 teaspoons mixed spice

1 teaspoon ground cinnamon

3 tablespoons canola oil

200 g vanilla yoghurt (gluten-free if on a gluten-free diet)

2 eggs

2 ripe bananas, mashed

1 cup (220 g) brown sugar

butter, to serve (optional)

Sweet chestnut cake

SERVES 8-12

This is a great cake for people with nut allergies as chestnuts are not actually nuts! Chestnut flour is available from gourmet food stores. Chestnut meal or natural almond meal may be used instead if you prefer a grainier texture.

Preheat the oven to 180°C. Grease a 24 cm springform tin and dust with gluten-free cornflour.

Sift the rice flour, cornflour, baking powder, bicarbonate of soda and xanthan gum three times into a bowl (or mix well with a whisk to ensure they are well combined).

Place the egg yolks and half the sugar in a medium bowl and beat with electric beaters for 5–6 minutes or until thick, creamy and doubled in volume. Gently beat in the yoghurt, oil and vanilla, then fold in the sifted flours and chestnut flour with a metal spoon.

Beat the egg whites in a clean bowl until soft peaks form. Add the remaining sugar and beat until stiff peaks form. Gently fold half the egg whites through the chestnut mixture, then fold in the remaining egg whites.

Pour the batter into the tin and bake for about 1 hour or until golden brown (a skewer inserted into the centre should come out clean). Cover with foil halfway through to prevent overbrowning. Remove from the oven and leave to cool in the tin for 10 minutes before transferring to a wire rack to cool completely. Dust with icing sugar and serve with cream, if liked.

½ cup (65 g) fine rice flour
½ cup (75 g) maize cornflour
2 teaspoons baking powder
   (gluten-free if on a gluten-free diet)
1 teaspoon bicarbonate of soda
1 teaspoon xanthan gum
6 eggs, separated
1 cup (220 g) caster sugar
200 g vanilla yoghurt (gluten-free
   if on a gluten-free diet)
½ cup (125 ml) canola oil
1 teaspoon vanilla essence
1 cup (145 g) chestnut flour
pure icing sugar, for dusting
cream, to serve (optional)

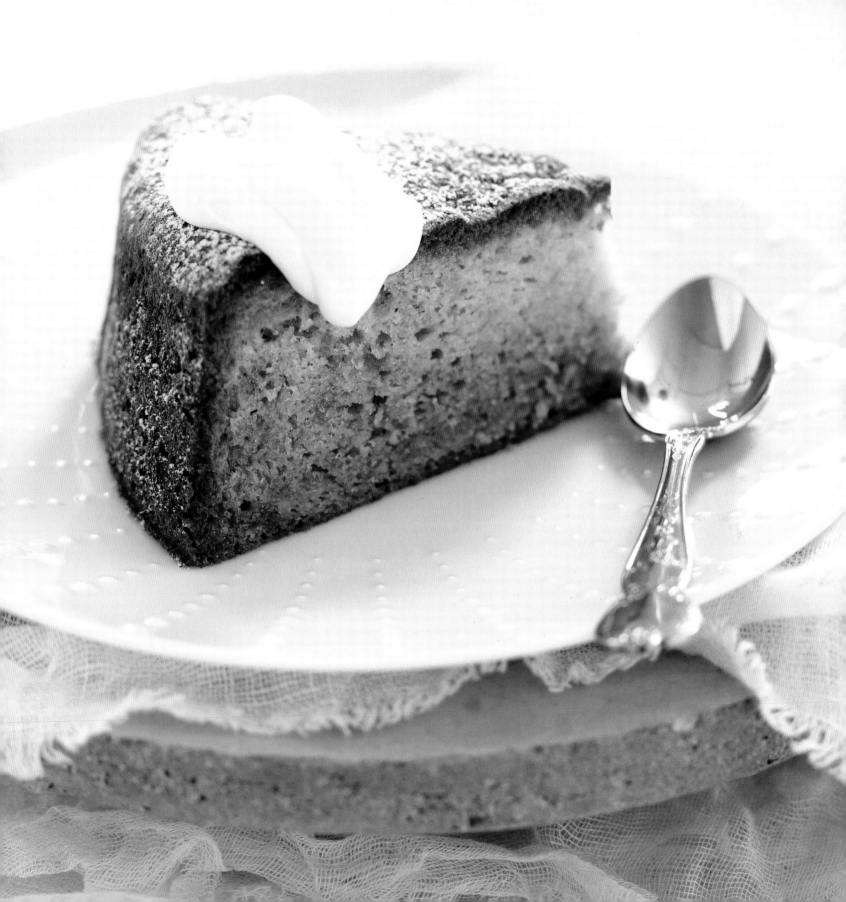

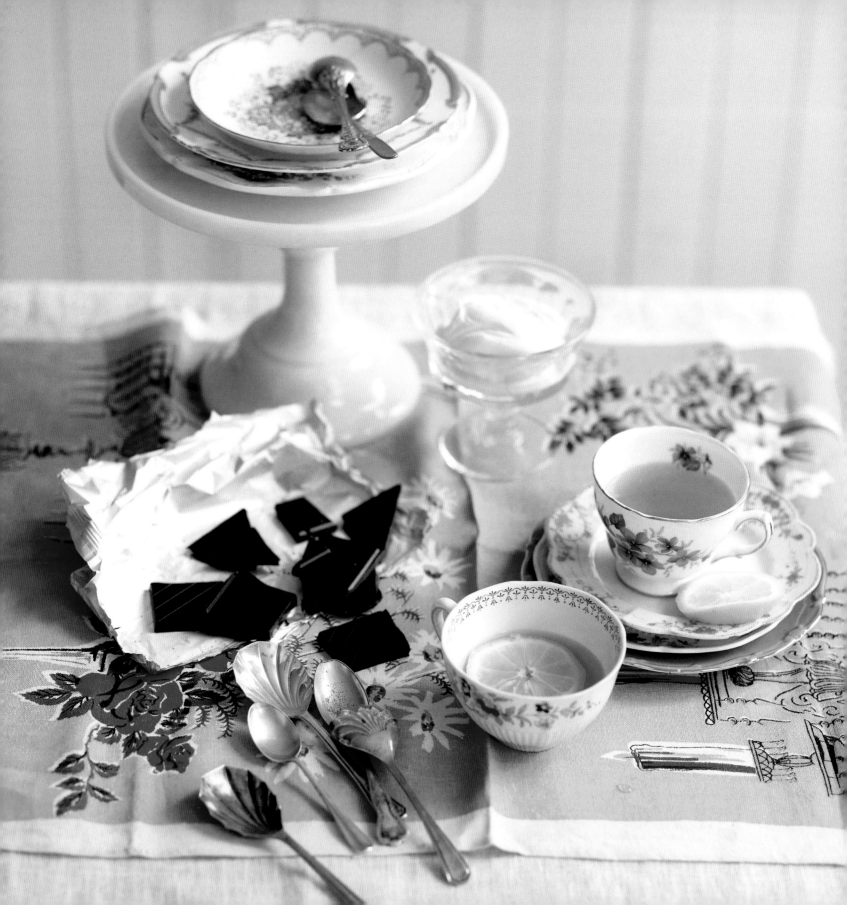

Desserts

Gooey chocolate puddings

SERVES 6

If you don't have ceramic ramekins, you can use large Texas muffin tins for these decadent puddings. For a final flourish, serve them with fresh strawberries and thick cream.

Preheat the oven to 180°C. Grease six ⅔ cup (175 ml) ramekins.

Place the chocolate and butter in a small saucepan and stir over low heat for 5 minutes or until smooth and completely melted. Leave to cool for 5 minutes.

Beat the eggs, egg yolks and brown sugar with electric beaters for 5–10 minutes or until doubled in volume. Fold in the cooled chocolate with a metal spoon. Sprinkle the rice flour over the mixture and gently fold through.

Spoon the batter into the ramekins. Place on a baking tray and bake for 10 minutes or until just firm to touch.

Meanwhile, to make the sauce, place the chocolate and cream in a small saucepan over medium–low heat and stir until the chocolate has melted and the sauce is smooth and well combined. Stir in the icing sugar.

Turn out the puddings onto individual plates or just serve in the ramekins. Drizzle with the chocolate sauce and serve warm.

200 g dark chocolate

150 g unsalted butter, chopped

4 eggs, at room temperature

4 egg yolks, at room temperature

½ cup (110 g) brown sugar

40 g fine rice flour

CHOCOLATE SAUCE

200 g dark chocolate

1 cup (250 ml) pouring cream

3 tablespoons pure icing sugar

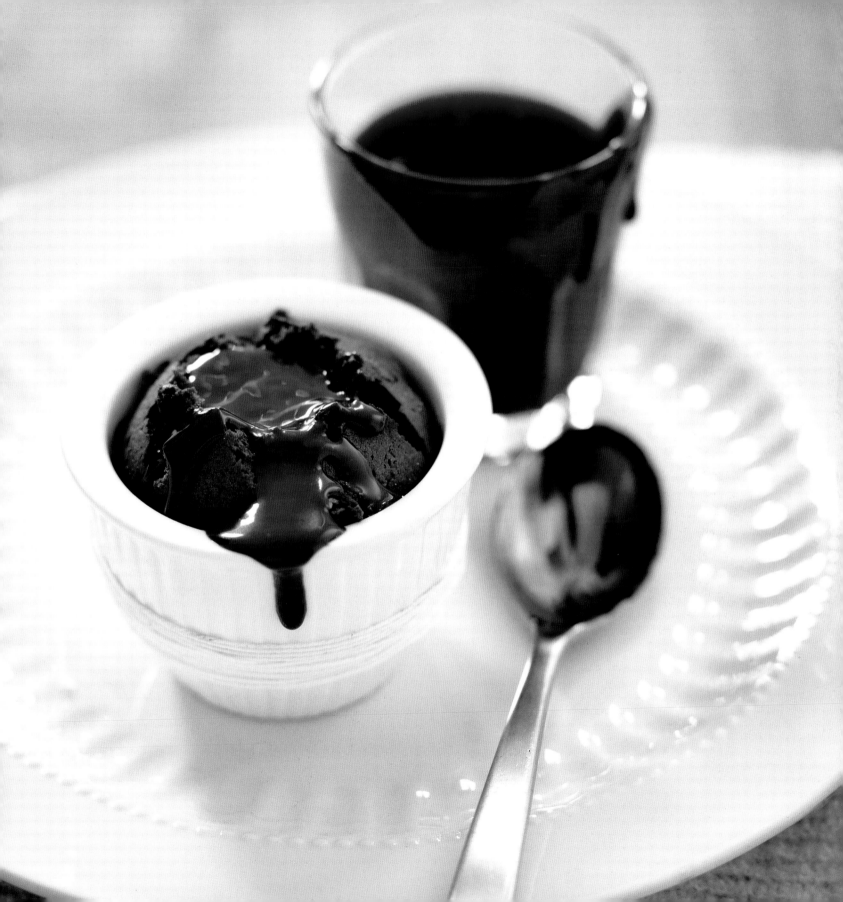

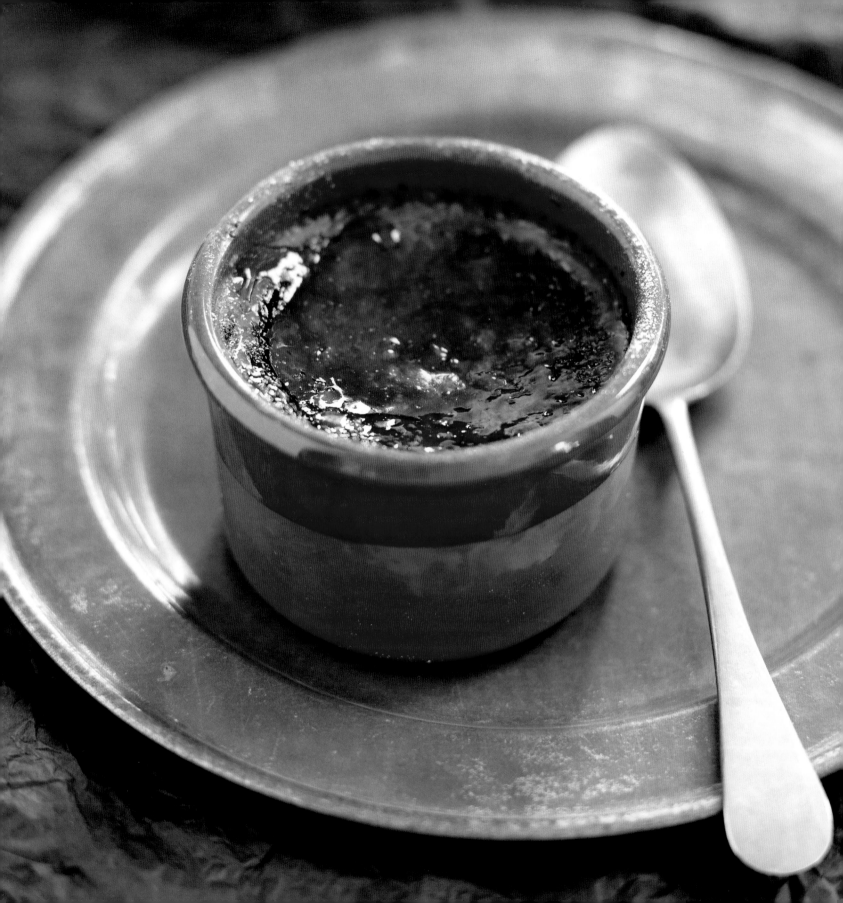

Cinnamon chilli chocolate brulees

SERVES 6

Now here's an interesting combination: rich creamy chocolate pots with a surprise chilli kick. If you prefer a gentle nudge of chilli, reduce the quantity to just a pinch. Note that you need to start preparing this dish the day before serving.

Preheat the oven to 150°C. Place six ½ cup (125 ml) ramekins in a baking dish.

Place the cream, chocolate, cinnamon and chilli in a medium saucepan and stir over medium heat until smooth and the chocolate has melted. Remove from the heat and cool to room temperature.

Beat the egg yolks and ⅓ cup (75 g) sugar with electric beaters until pale and creamy. Add the cooled chocolate mixture and beat until well combined.

Divide the mixture among the ramekins, then pour enough boiling water into the baking dish to come halfway up the sides of the ramekins. Bake on the lowest shelf of the oven for 45–50 minutes or until firm around the edges.

Remove the ramekins from the baking dish and set aside to cool to room temperature (this will take about an hour). Cover with plastic film and place in the fridge for 8 hours or overnight to set.

Sprinkle the remaining sugar over the brulees and place under a hot grill for about a minute until the sugar bubbles and caramelises. (Alternatively, use a kitchen blowtorch to do this.) Set aside for 5 minutes before serving.

600 ml thickened cream
125 g dark couverture chocolate
2 teaspoons ground cinnamon
¼ teaspoon chilli powder
6 egg yolks
½ cup (110 g) caster sugar

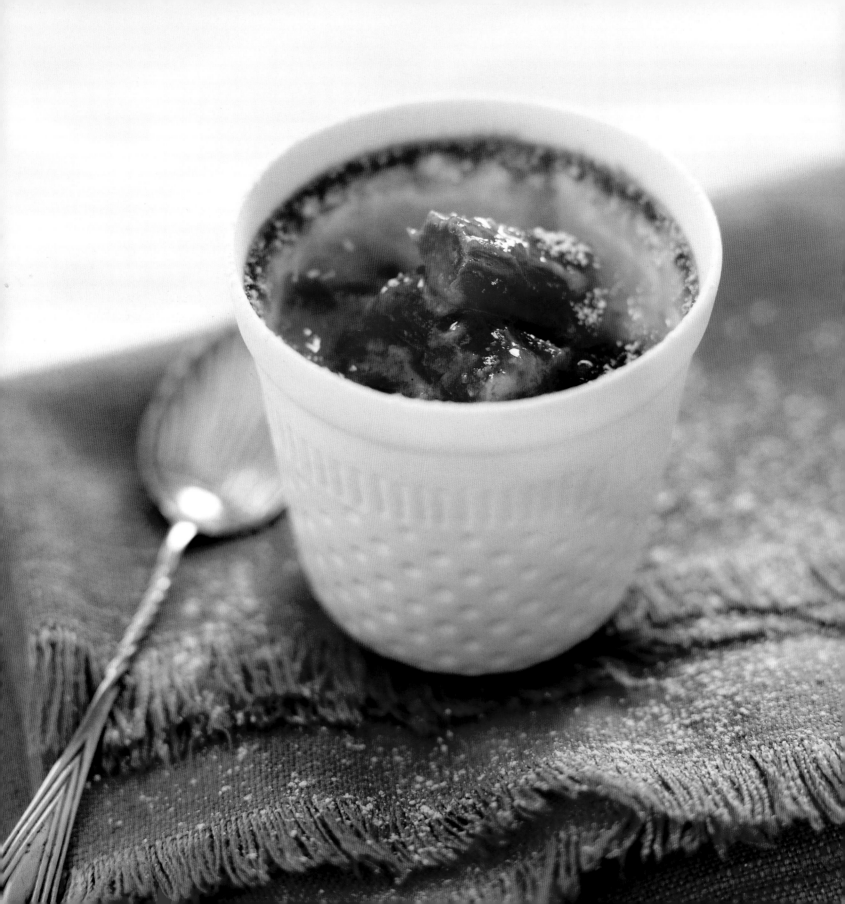

Dairy-free baked rhubarb custards

MAKES 6

This recipe suits those following the Low-FODMAP Diet, and is also dairy free. The unique flavour of rhubarb tastes great in this delicious dessert, but stewed berries would also work well.

Preheat the oven to 180°C and grease six 1 cup (250 ml) ramekins.

Bring a large saucepan of water to the boil. Add the rhubarb and half the sugar and cook over medium–high heat for 7–8 minutes or until the rhubarb has softened. Drain and discard the liquid. Spoon the rhubarb evenly into the ramekins, then place the ramekins in a baking dish.

Combine the rice milk and vanilla in a small saucepan and bring to the boil. Reduce the heat and simmer for 5–10 minutes, stirring regularly.

Whisk together the egg yolks and remaining sugar in a heatproof jug. Slowly pour in the warm rice milk, whisking constantly, then strain through a fine sieve into a clean saucepan. Heat over medium–low heat for 5 minutes or until the custard simmers and starts to thicken.

Pour the custard over the rhubarb in the ramekins, then pour enough boiling water into the baking dish to come halfway up the sides of the ramekins. Bake on the lowest shelf of the oven for 30–35 minutes or until just firm. Remove the ramekins from the baking dish and set aside to cool for 5 minutes. Dust with icing sugar and serve immediately.

5 rhubarb stalks, well washed
    and cut into 2 cm lengths
1 cup (220 g) caster sugar
2 cups (500 ml) rice milk (gluten-free
    if on a gluten-free diet)
2 teaspoons vanilla bean paste
    (or 1 vanilla bean)
6 egg yolks
pure icing sugar, for dusting

Panna cotta with rosewater cinnamon syrup

SERVES 4

Rosewater is probably best known as the flavour base in Turkish Delight. Here, it is combined with cinnamon to make this light, creamy dessert something really special.

Grease four ½ cup (125 ml) dariole moulds.

Place the cream, milk, sugar and vanilla bean paste in a small saucepan over low heat and cook, stirring regularly, for 20 minutes or until the mixture has thickened enough to coat the back of a spoon (do not allow it to boil). Remove from the heat.

Combine the gelatine and 1 tablespoon boiling water in a small heatproof bowl. Set the bowl over a larger bowl of boiling water and stir constantly until all the gelatine has dissolved. Whisk into the custard, then pour into a medium bowl.

Fill a large bowl with ice cubes. Sit the bowl of custard on top of the ice-filled bowl and whisk every few minutes for about 10 minutes until thickened enough to coat the back of a wooden spoon. Pour into the moulds and refrigerate for 2–3 hours.

Meanwhile, to make the syrup, combine the sugar, cinnamon and ⅓ cup (80 ml) water in a small saucepan over low heat and cook, stirring regularly, until the sugar has dissolved. Increase the heat to medium–high and bring to the boil, then reduce the heat and simmer gently for 5–7 minutes or until the liquid has reduced by half. Remove the pan from the heat, stir in the rosewater essence and leave to cool to room temperature.

To serve, dip each dariole mould in hot water for a few seconds, then turn out onto serving plates. Drizzle the cooled syrup over the top.

1⅔ cups (420 ml) reduced-fat cream
½ cup (125 ml) low-fat milk
½ cup (110 g) caster sugar
2 teaspoons vanilla bean paste
2¼ teaspoons gelatine powder

ROSEWATER CINNAMON SYRUP
75 g caster sugar
2 × 3 cm pieces cinnamon stick
1½ teaspoons rosewater essence

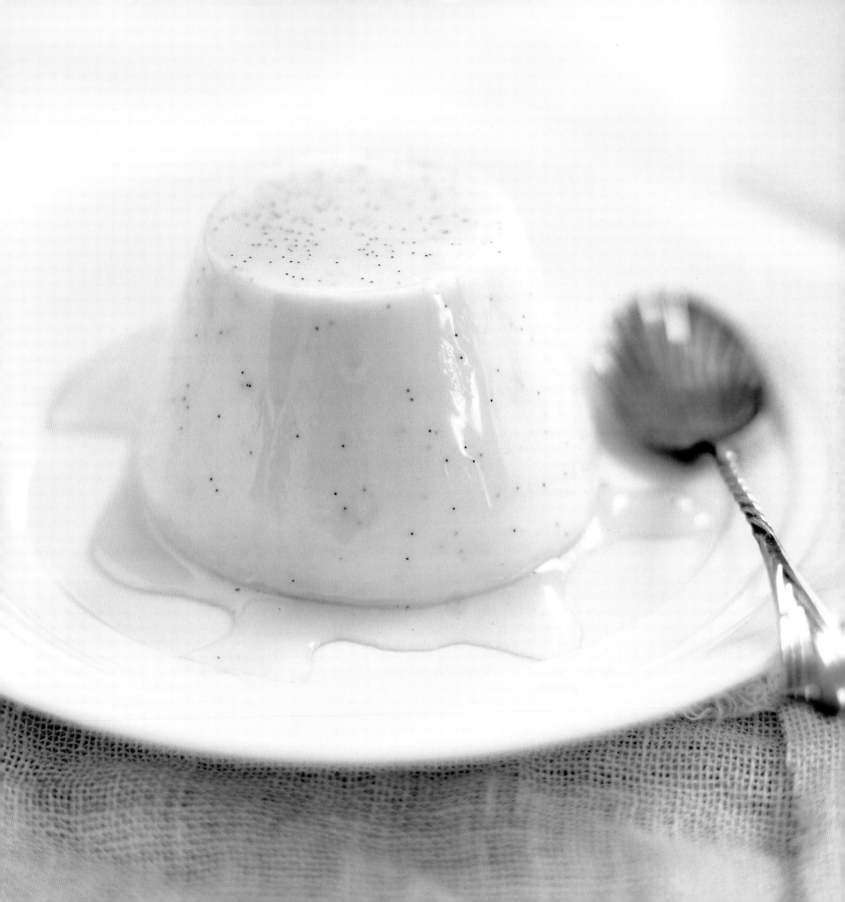

Baked caramel cheesecake

You may wish to use the sweet biscuit recipe on page 190 to make the base for this cheesecake; otherwise, look for plain, sweet gluten-free biscuits in supermarkets and health-food stores.

Grease a 20 cm springform tin.

Place the biscuits in a food processor and process to make crumbs. Add the melted butter and process until well combined. Press the mixture into the base of the tin, cover with plastic film and refrigerate for 30 minutes.

Preheat the oven to 150°C.

Beat the cream cheese, sugar and vanilla with electric beaters until well combined. Add the eggs one at a time, beating between additions, and then the egg yolk. Add the chopped caramel pieces and stir well with a metal spoon.

Pour the mixture into the tin over the biscuit base and bake for 1 hour or until just firm to touch. Turn the oven off and leave the cheesecake in the oven with the door ajar for 4 hours or until cooled completely. This prevents the cheesecake from cracking. When cool, cover with plastic film and refrigerate for at least 2 hours before serving. Dust with icing sugar, if liked.

200 g plain sweet gluten-free biscuits

110 g unsalted butter, melted

500 g cream cheese, at room temperature

⅔ cup (150 g) caster sugar

2 teaspoons vanilla extract

3 eggs

1 egg yolk

250 g chewy caramel confectionery (gluten-free if on a gluten-free diet), chopped into 1 cm cubes

pure icing sugar, for dusting (optional)

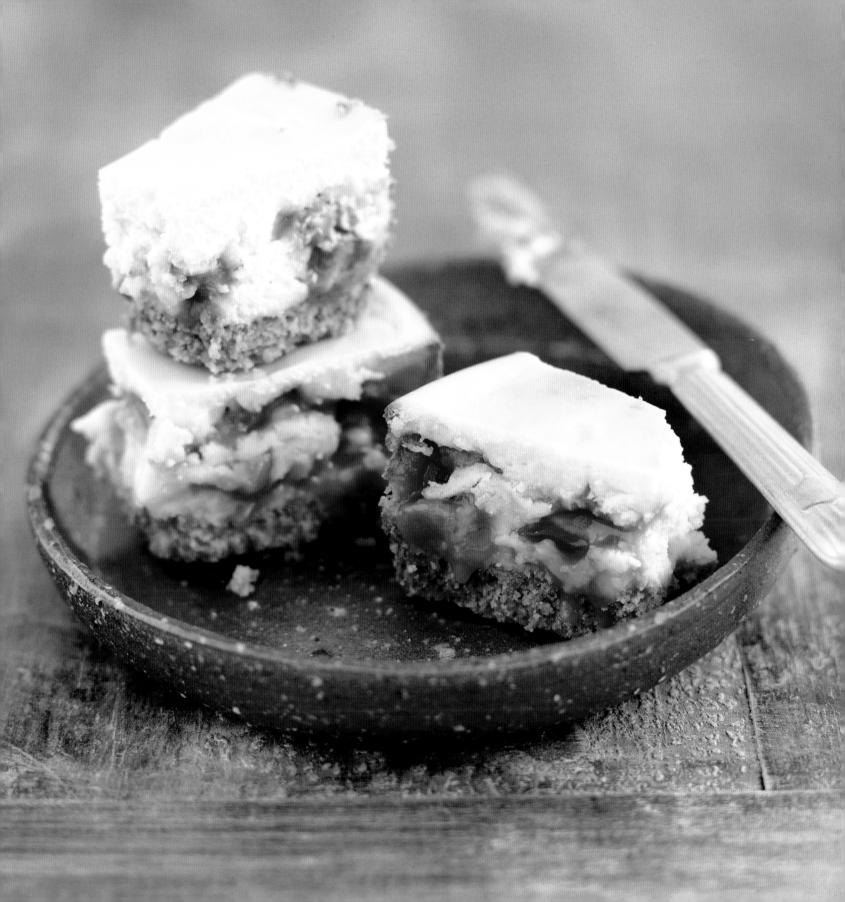

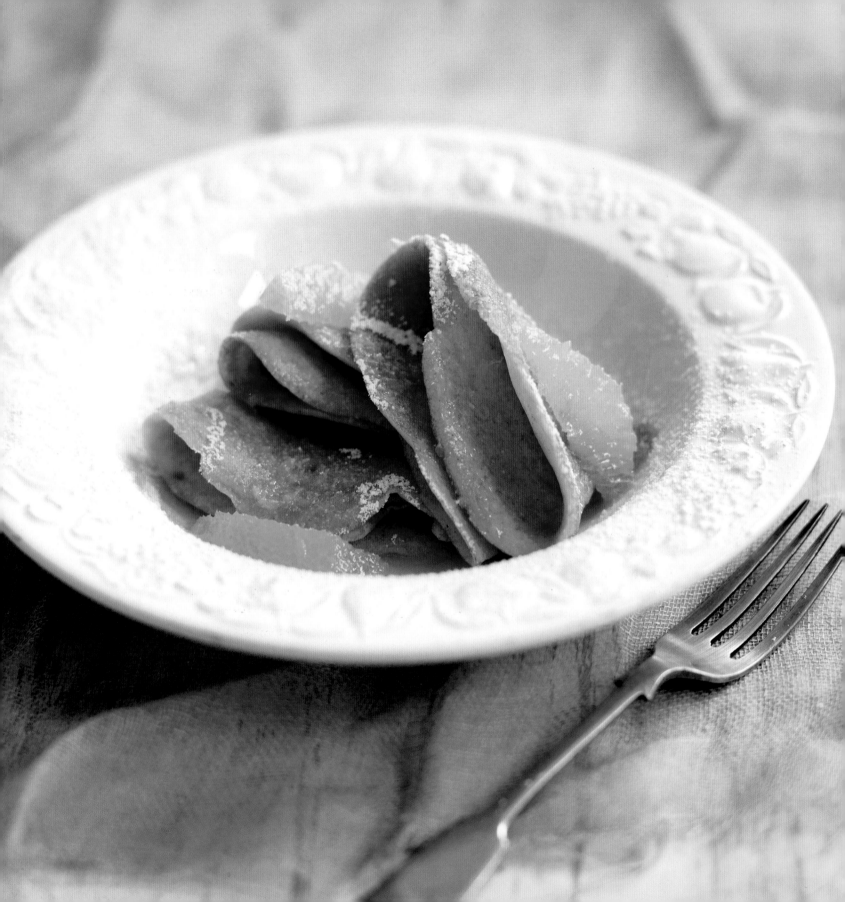

Crepes suzette

SERVES 4

This is the Low-FODMAP Diet version of what is probably the most famous crepe dish in the world. Traditionally, brandy is poured over the crepes then lit so the dessert is flaming when served, but I generally leave this step out! The amount of soy flour used in the recipe is minimal so it will suit most people following the Low-FODMAP Diet. Assess your individual tolerance – if necessary, replace the soy flour with tapioca flour.

Sift the flours and bicarbonate of soda three times into a large bowl (or mix well with a whisk to ensure they are well combined). Make a well in the middle, add the beaten egg, milk, sugar and orange zest and blend with a spoon to form a smooth batter. Stir in the melted butter. Cover with plastic film and set aside for 20 minutes.

Heat an 18 cm non-stick frying pan over medium heat and spray with cooking spray. Pour 3–4 tablespoons batter into the pan and tilt to coat the base. Cook until bubbles start to appear, then turn and cook the other side. Remove to a plate and cover with foil to keep warm. Repeat with the remaining batter to make eight crepes in all.

To make the sauce, place the orange juice, zest, sugar and liqueur in a small bowl and mix well. Melt the butter in the crepe pan over low heat, then slowly add the orange mixture and heat gently.

Place one crepe in the pan and warm through. Fold it in half, and then in half again to make a wedge shape. Tilt the pan to flow all the sauce away from the crepe, then remove the crepe and set aside on a warmed plate. Cover with foil. Repeat with the remaining crepes and serve warm with the remaining sauce drizzled over the top. Serve with orange segments and dust with icing sugar, if desired.

¾ cup (130 g) rice flour

½ cup (75 g) maize cornflour

⅓ cup (30 g) debittered soy flour

¾ teaspoon bicarbonate of soda

2 eggs, lightly beaten

2 cups (500 ml) low-fat milk

2 tablespoons caster sugar

1 tablespoon grated orange zest

40 g butter, melted

cooking spray

orange segments, to serve

pure icing sugar, for dusting (optional)

SUZETTE SAUCE

1 cup (250 ml) orange juice

grated zest of 2 oranges

grated zest of 1 small lemon

1 teaspoon caster sugar
  (more if desired)

4 tablespoons Grand Marnier
  or Cointreau

80 g butter

Caramel banana sago puddings

SERVES 6

Cooked sago balls, often called sago pearls, are the base for these soft, creamy puddings. People with lactose intolerance should use lactose-free milk.

Place the milk, vanilla and brown sugar in a medium saucepan and bring to the boil over medium–high heat, stirring well. Reduce the heat to low and stir in the sago. Simmer gently, stirring regularly, for 30–35 minutes or until the sago is soft and resembles translucent jelly-like balls. Set aside to cool for 5–10 minutes.

  In a small bowl, mix the mashed banana with half the extra brown sugar. Stir through the cooked sago, then pour the mixture evenly into six ½ cup (125 ml) ceramic dessert moulds. Sprinkle with the rest of the brown sugar and refrigerate for 3–4 hours or until set.

1 litre low-fat milk
2 teaspoons vanilla extract
60 g brown sugar
⅓ cup (65 g) sago
2 ripe bananas, mashed with a fork
⅓ cup (75 g) brown sugar, extra

Warm bananas in sweet citrus sauce

SERVES 4

This simple, dairy-free dessert makes a delicious conclusion to any meal. The rum is optional, and Grand Marnier or Cointreau could also be used.

Place the butter and brown sugar in a medium frying pan over medium–high heat and cook until the butter is golden brown.

  Mix the cornflour with a little orange juice to form a paste. Stir in the rum (if using) and remaining orange juice. Pour into the pan, stir well and bring to a gentle simmer.

  Cut the bananas into large pieces on the diagonal. Add to the pan and fry on both sides until golden brown. Divide the bananas and sauce among four bowls and serve with ice cream.

2 teaspoons unsalted butter
2 tablespoons brown sugar
1 teaspoon maize cornflour
juice of 2 oranges
1 tablespoon rum (optional)
4 large firm bananas
vanilla ice cream, to serve

Caramel banana sago puddings →

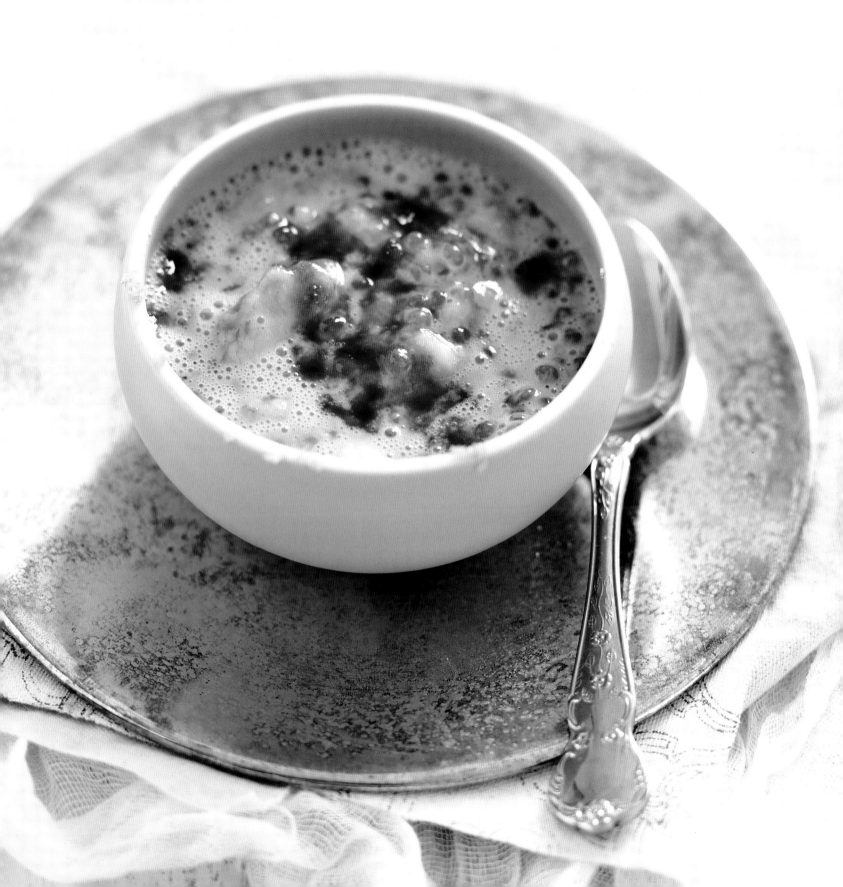

Golden syrup puddings

SERVES 6

These delicious puddings are warm and comforting, and make a nice change from chocolate. You can also add chopped macadamias or pecans for a bit of crunch. To make one large pudding, use an 18 cm square baking dish and increase the cooking time to 40–45 minutes.

Preheat the oven to 160°C and grease six 1 cup (250 ml) ovenproof dishes.

Place the butter and golden syrup in a small saucepan and stir over medium–high heat until combined and the butter has melted. Pour into the dishes.

Sift the flours, bicarbonate of soda, baking powder and xanthan gum three times into a large bowl (or mix well with a whisk to ensure they are well combined). Add the sugar, milk, egg and vanilla and beat with electric beaters until well combined.

Dollop small balls of the batter over the golden syrup mixture in the dishes until evenly covered. Sprinkle with the extra sugar and bake for 30–35 minutes or until golden and cooked through. Leave for 5 minutes before serving with cream or custard.

125 g unsalted butter
½ cup (125 ml) golden syrup
1 cup (130 g) fine rice flour
½ cup (75 g) maize cornflour
½ cup (90 g) potato flour
1 teaspoon bicarbonate of soda
2 teaspoons baking powder
    (gluten-free if on a gluten-free diet)
1 teaspoon xanthan gum
1 cup (220 g) sugar
¾ cup (185 ml) low-fat milk
1 egg
2 teaspoons vanilla extract
3 tablespoons sugar, extra
cream or custard, to serve

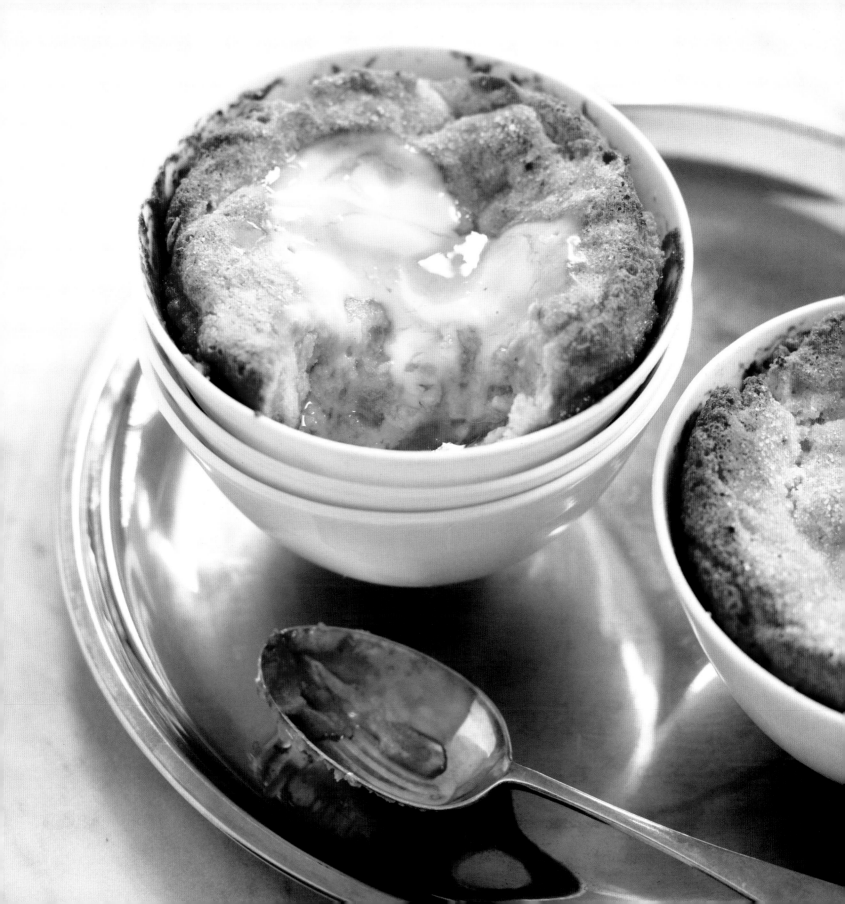

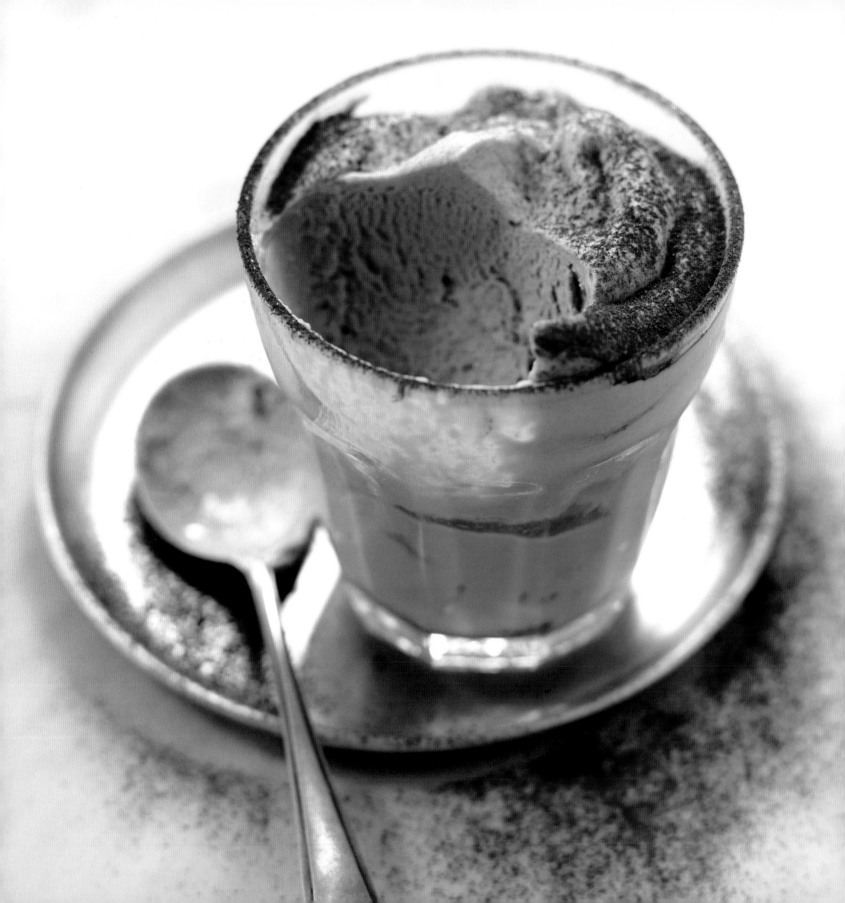

Frozen cappuccino

SERVES 6

This ice-cream recipe makes enough for six good-size portions, but I often use it to make eight smaller serves – there is still enough mixture to ensure everyone gets a satisfying share! If you are lactose intolerant, limit yourself to a half-serve.

4 egg whites

200 g caster sugar

2 tablespoons instant coffee

⅔ cup (170 ml) pouring cream

180 g mascarpone

cocoa powder, for dusting (optional)

Beat the egg whites and half the sugar until stiff peaks form.

Combine the coffee, remaining sugar and ⅓ cup (80 ml) water in a small saucepan and stir over medium–high heat until the mixture is bubbling and syrupy. If you have a sugar thermometer, it should be heated to 120°C.

Slowly pour the coffee syrup into the egg whites and beat until well combined. Cover with plastic film and refrigerate until completely cold.

Beat the cream with electric beaters until firm peaks form, then gently fold in the mascarpone with a metal spoon. Fold in the cold coffee mixture until well combined. Pour into six 200 ml dessert bowls, glasses or small coffee cups and freeze for 4 hours. Take out of the freezer 5 minutes before serving. Dust with cocoa powder, if desired.

Strawberry slice

MAKES 20 PIECES

You could also use strawberry jelly crystals (made according to the packet directions but using half the quantity of water) to top this delicious slice in place of the pureed strawberries. For people who are lactose intolerant, use lactose-free milk.

Line a 22 cm square baking dish with baking paper.

Combine the butter and brown sugar in a medium saucepan and stir over medium–low heat until the butter has melted and the sugar has dissolved. Add the egg and stir until thickened. Add the biscuit crumbs and mix well. Press into the base of the baking dish and set aside.

To make the filling, mix the cornflour with a little milk to make a smooth paste. Gradually add the cream and remaining milk and stir to combine. Add the sugar and vanilla and heat gently over medium heat, stirring regularly with a wooden spoon, until the mixture is smooth and thick. Remove the pan from the heat and beat in the egg yolk. Set aside to cool for 5–10 minutes. Stir in the chopped strawberries, then pour the custard mixture over the prepared base. Refrigerate for 3–4 hours or until firm and cooled through.

To make the topping, place the strawberries in a food processor and puree until smooth. Combine the boiling water and gelatine in a small heatproof bowl. Set the bowl over a larger bowl of boiling water, stirring constantly until the gelatine has dissolved. Stir into the pureed strawberries.

Remove the dish from the fridge and pour the strawberry topping over the custard filling. Return to the fridge for a further 2–3 hours or until the topping has set firm. Use a hot knife to cut into pieces.

80 g unsalted butter

½ cup (110 g) brown sugar

1 egg, beaten

200 g plain sweet gluten-free biscuits (see page 190), crushed

FILLING

½ cup (75 g) maize cornflour

2 cups (500 ml) milk

¾ cup (185 ml) pouring cream

80 g caster sugar

2 teaspoons vanilla extract

2 egg yolks

100 g strawberries, hulled and chopped

TOPPING

200 g strawberries, hulled

3 tablespoons boiling water

2 teaspoons powdered gelatine

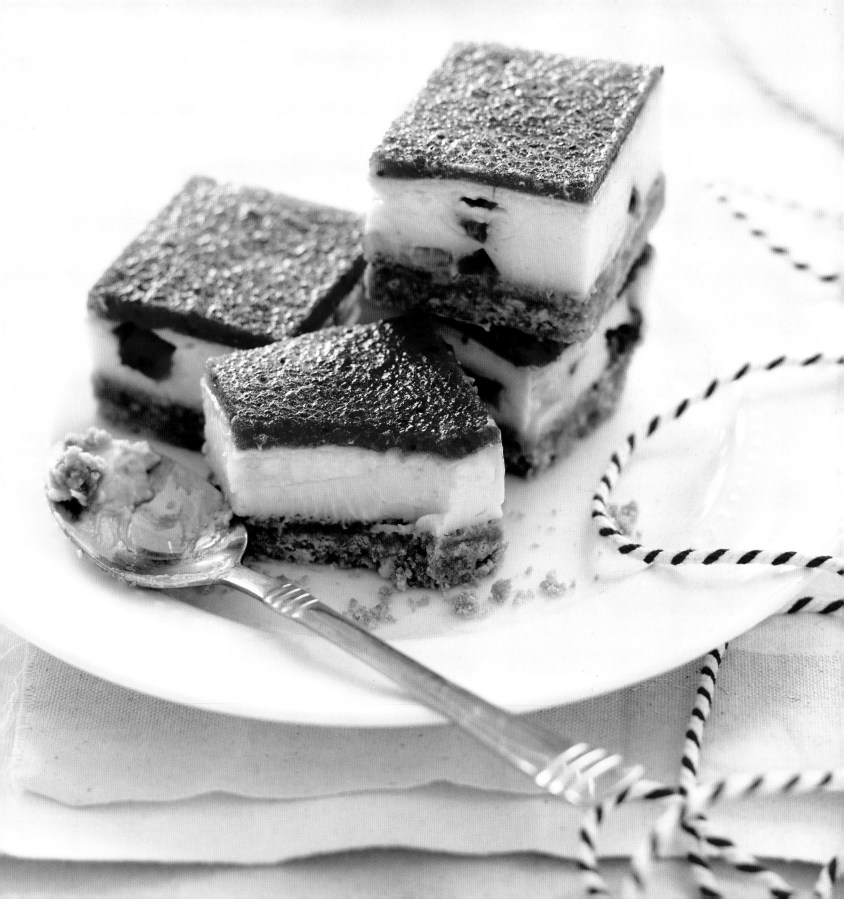

Baked ricotta with stewed spiced rhubarb

SERVES 8–10

This is a great dinner party dessert. Unfortunately, it is not suitable for people with lactose intolerance (unless you can limit yourself to a very small serve!).

Preheat the oven to 140°C. Grease and line a 25 cm × 11 cm loaf tin with baking paper.

Beat the ricotta, flours, sugar and vanilla with electric beaters for about 2–3 minutes or until well combined. Add the eggs one at a time, beating well between additions.

Pour the mixture into the tin and bake for 40–45 minutes or until a skewer inserted into the centre comes out clean. Turn the oven off and leave the ricotta to cool in the oven with the door ajar for about 2 hours. Remove from the oven and leave to cool completely in the tin.

To make the stewed rhubarb, place the rhubarb and sugar in a medium saucepan, cover with water and cook over medium heat for 8–10 minutes or until just tender. Drain, reserving the liquid. Stir the mixed spice and extra sugar through the rhubarb while still warm.

To serve, cut the baked ricotta into 4 cm thick slices, then cut into fingers. Arrange on serving plates with a spoonful of spiced rhubarb on the side. Drizzle with the reserved cooking liquid and serve.

1 kg fresh ricotta

3 tablespoons fine rice flour

2 tablespoons maize cornflour

½ cup (110 g) caster sugar

1 tablespoon vanilla extract

6 eggs

STEWED SPICED RHUBARB

500 g rhubarb stalks,
   cut into 3 cm pieces

½ cup (110 g) caster sugar

2 teaspoons mixed spice

3 tablespoons caster sugar, extra

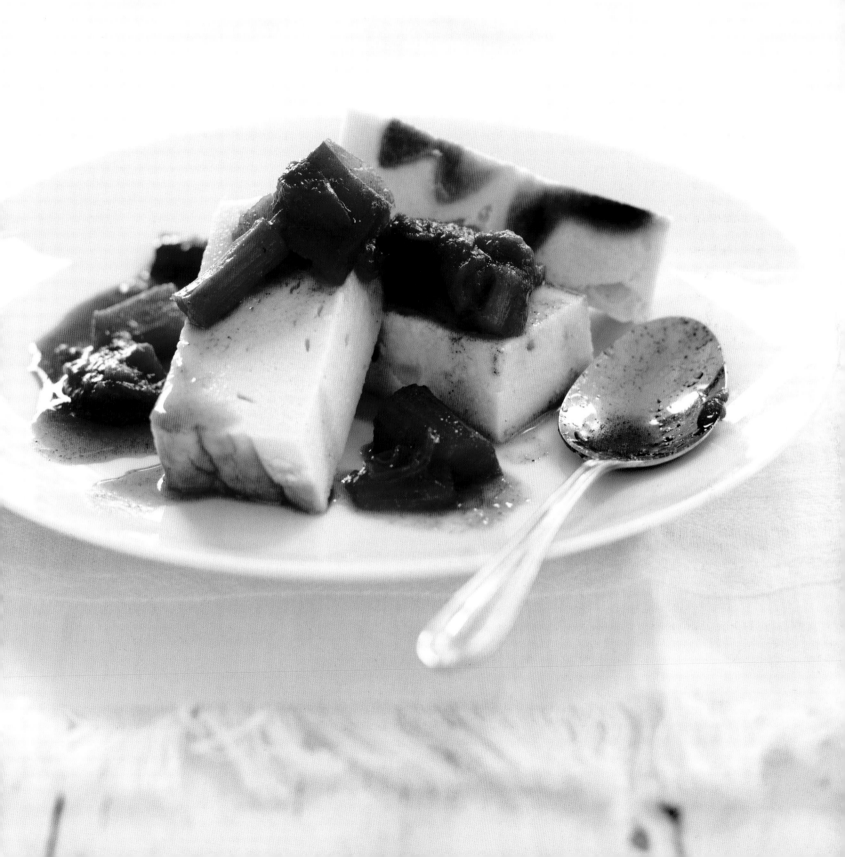

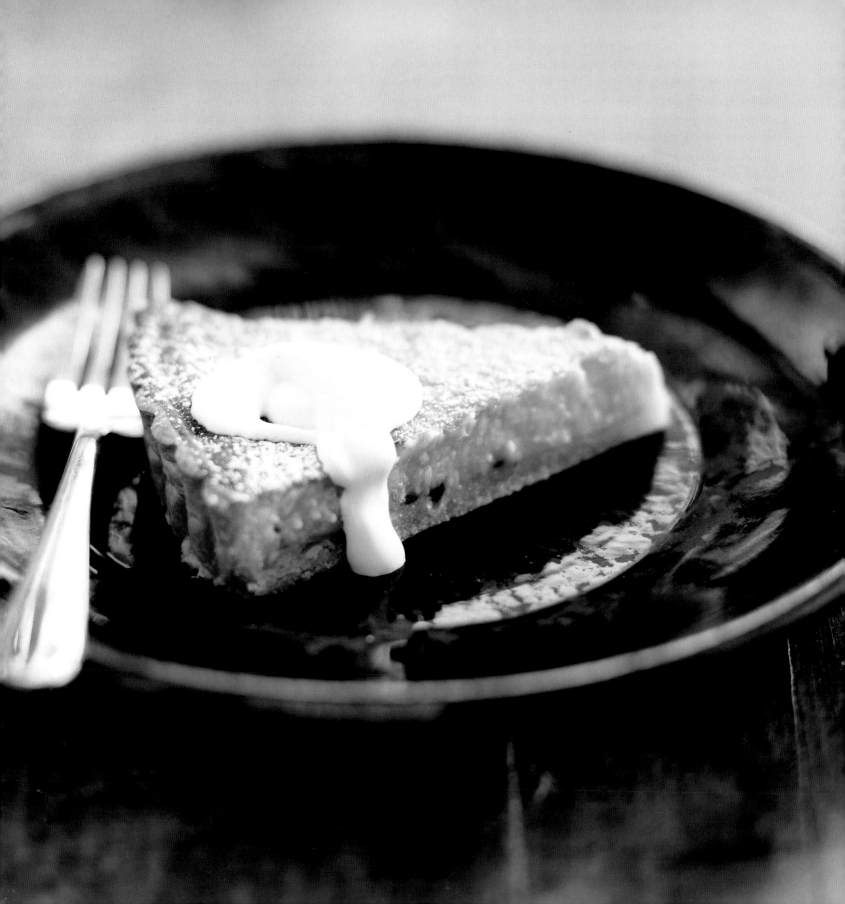

Passionfruit tart

SERVES 8–10

I love the fresh flavours of this passionfruit tart. The trick to making the pastry is to add the water one tablespoon at a time – stop as soon as the desired consistency is achieved. Depending on the temperature in your kitchen, you may not need all the water specified. The amount of soy flour used in this recipe is minimal so it will suit most people following the Low-FODMAP Diet. Assess your individual tolerance.

Preheat the oven to 170°C. Grease a 23 cm fluted tart dish with a removable base.

To make the pastry, sift the flours and xanthan gum three times into a bowl (or mix well with a whisk to ensure they are well combined). Transfer to a food processor, add the sugar and butter and process until the mixture resembles fine breadcrumbs. While the motor is running, add the iced water (a tablespoon at a time) to form a soft dough. You may not need all the water. Turn out onto a bench dusted with gluten-free cornflour and knead until smooth. Wrap in plastic film and refrigerate for 30 minutes.

Bring the dough to room temperature, then place between two sheets of baking paper and roll out to a thickness of 3–5 mm. Ease the pastry into the tart dish and trim the edges to neaten. Line the pastry case with baking paper, fill with baking beads or rice and blind-bake for 10–15 minutes or until lightly golden. Remove the paper and beads or rice.

Beat the sugar, passionfruit pulp and mascarpone in a small bowl. Add the eggs one at a time, beating well between additions. Pour into the pastry case and bake for 1 hour or until set and a skewer inserted into the centre comes out clean. Cool to room temperature and dust with icing sugar. Serve with cream, if desired.

⅔ cup (150 g) caster sugar
170 g tin passionfruit in syrup
150 g mascarpone
3 eggs
pure icing sugar, for dusting
cream, to serve (optional)

PASTRY

1 cup (130 g) fine rice flour
½ cup (75 g) maize cornflour
½ cup (45 g) debittered soy flour
1 teaspoon xanthan gum
3 tablespoons caster sugar
160 g unsalted butter, chopped
80–120 ml iced water

New York cheesecake

SERVES 8–10

It is hard to resist going back for seconds (and thirds) of this classic dessert. It's gorgeous on its own, but can also be dressed up with whipped cream and fresh raspberries. People with lactose intolerance can enjoy it by replacing the cream cheese with soy cream cheese.

Grease and line a 22 cm springform tin with baking paper. Crush the biscuits in a food processor and add the melted butter. Combine well, then press into the base and side of the tin. Cover with plastic film and refrigerate for 1 hour.

Preheat the oven to 160°C.

Beat the cream cheese, sugar, vanilla, lemon zest and cornflour with electric beaters until well combined. Add the eggs one at a time, beating well between additions. Pour in the cream and mix until just combined.

Pour the cream cheese mixture over the biscuit base. Bake for 1¼–1½ hours or until just set in the centre (it should be firm when gently shaken). Turn the oven off and leave the cheesecake to cool in the oven with the door ajar for about 2 hours. Place in the refrigerator to cool completely. Decorate with the raspberries and dust with icing sugar before serving.

200 g plain sweet gluten-free biscuits (see page 190)
100 g unsalted butter, melted
750 g cream cheese, at room temperature
1 cup (220 g) caster sugar
2 teaspoons vanilla extract
2 teaspoons finely grated lemon zest
2 tablespoons maize cornflour
4 eggs
300 ml thickened cream
fresh raspberries, to serve
pure icing sugar, for dusting

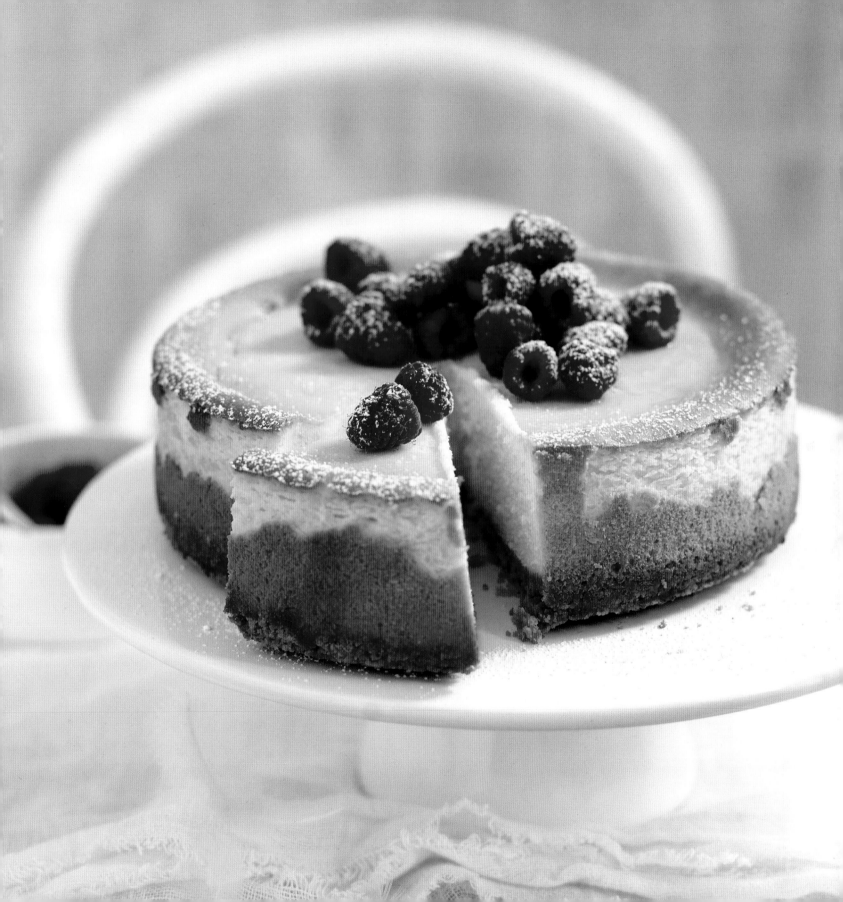

Polenta dessert cake with lime and strawberry syrup

SERVES 10–12

The polenta and ground almonds give a pleasing grainy texture to this delectable cake. The lime and strawberry combination may seem a little unusual, but you'll love its delicious freshness. The cake may be served warm or at room temperature.

Preheat the oven to 160°C. Grease and line a 20 cm springform tin with baking paper.

Beat the egg yolks, eggs and sugar until thick and pale. Stir in the vanilla and lime zest. Combine the ground almonds, flour, polenta and baking powder in a small bowl, then fold into the egg mixture with a metal spoon. Add the melted butter and stir to combine.

Pour the mixture into the cake tin and bake for 45–55 minutes or until a skewer inserted into the centre comes out clean. Cover with foil halfway through to prevent overbrowning. Remove from the oven and allow to cool in the tin for 10 minutes before transferring to a wire rack to cool completely.

To make the syrup, place the lime zest, juice, sugar and ½ cup (125 ml) water in a medium saucepan and stir over medium heat until the sugar has dissolved. Bring the mixture to the boil, then reduce the heat to low and add the strawberries. Simmer gently for 10–15 minutes until the syrup has thickened and the strawberries have softened.

Cut the cake into slices and serve with a generous spoonful of lime and strawberry syrup.

5 egg yolks

2 large eggs

1 cup (220 g) caster sugar

2 teaspoons vanilla extract

grated zest of 2 limes

1 cup (120 g) ground almonds

90 g fine rice flour

75 g instant polenta

2 teaspoons baking powder
   (gluten-free if on a gluten-free diet)

150 g unsalted butter, melted

LIME AND STRAWBERRY SYRUP

grated zest and juice of 1 lime

120 g caster sugar

1 punnet (250 g) strawberries,
   hulled and thickly sliced

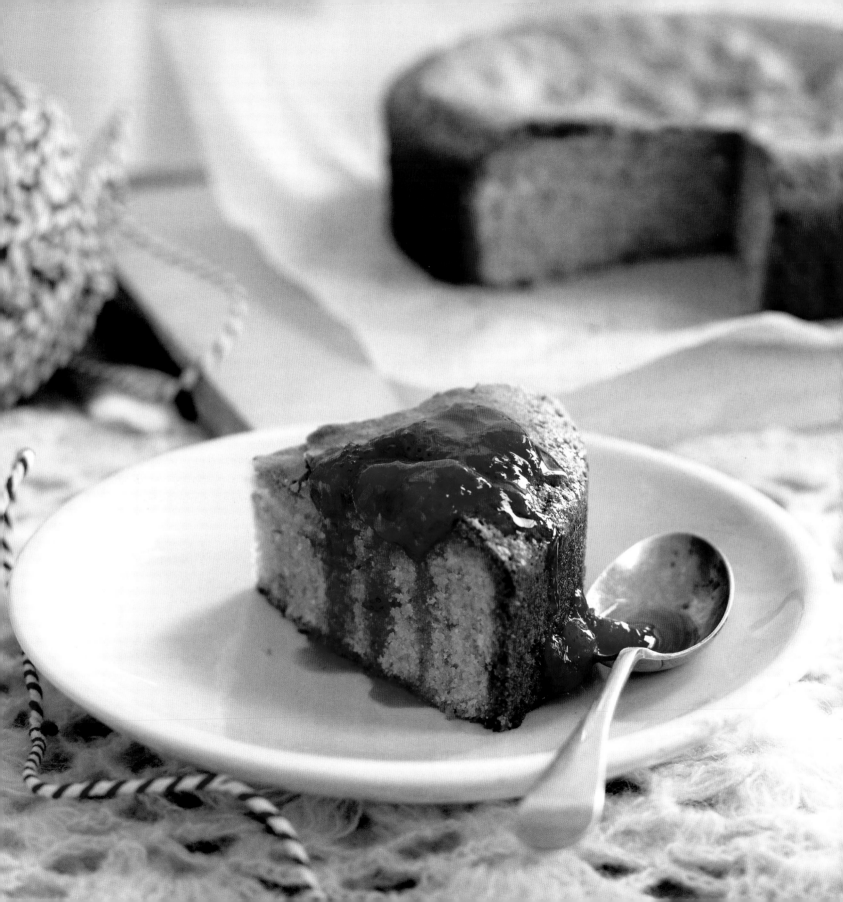

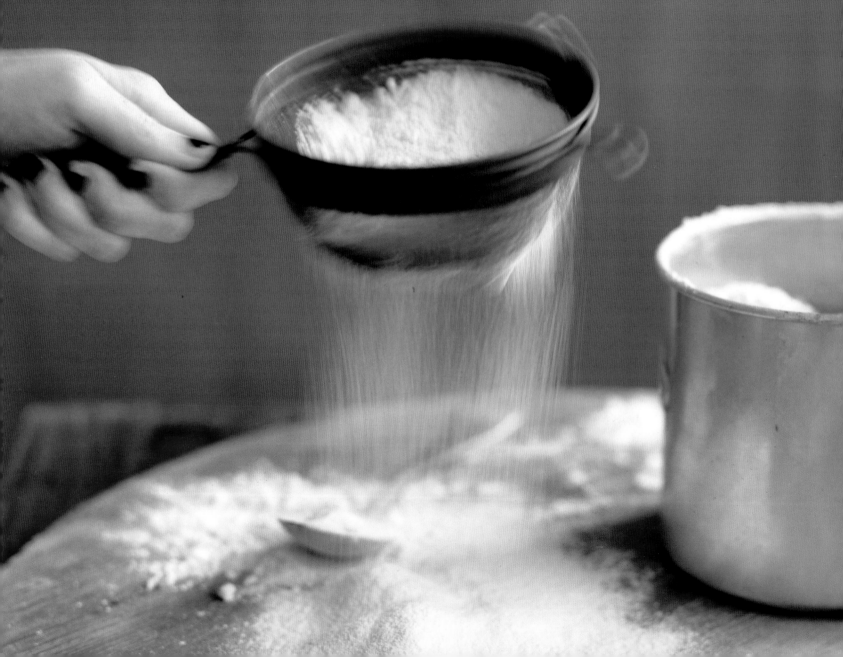

Flours and baking ingredients

BAKING POWDER

Baking powder is a raising agent. Not all baking powders are gluten-free – always check the label before buying. A simple recipe for baking powder is 1 teaspoon cream of tartar and ½ teaspoon bicarbonate of soda. This can be added to 1 cup of a wheat-free flour blend to make it 'self-raising'.

BUCKWHEAT

Despite its name, buckwheat is not related to wheat at all – it is actually a member of the rhubarb family. It has a strong nutty flavour and is often made into flour and used in recipes such as pancakes.

CORNFLOUR

Gluten-free cornflour must be made from maize (corn). In some countries (including Australia and New Zealand) flour made from wheat can be called cornflour, so check the label. It has little taste, is low in protein, and makes an excellent addition to a wheat-free flour blend. It is perfect for thickening sauces.

POTATO FLOUR

Made from potato starch, potato flour is virtually tasteless. It can be used to thicken sweet and savoury sauces; however, the sauce will become a little 'stretchy' or gel-like. It is great in a wheat-free flour blend, especially for cakes and muffins, and makes a good substitute for tapioca flour and arrowroot. It is available in Asian grocery stores.

QUINOA

Pronounced 'keen-wah', quinoa can be used in a variety of ways: as pasta and flour, and as the whole grain, it can be cooked like rice and used as a basis for salads or side dishes. It has a slightly bitter taste. Available from health-food shops.

RICE FLOUR

White rice flour is the main contributor to a wheat-free flour blend and is an essential addition to any wheat-free pantry. The texture ranges from gritty to fine – fine rice flour is preferable and is readily available in Asian grocery shops. It has a neutral taste and can be used as a thickener for sauces and gravy. Brown rice flour is also available and can be used in wheat-free baking to increase the fibre content.

SOY FLOUR

Soy flour is a high-protein flour made from soy beans. It can have a strong flavour, and is sometimes bitter. This bitterness decreases with cooking, but it is better to purchase debittered soy flour if possible. Soy flour is best used as a small part of a wheat-free flour blend. It is available from health-food shops.

TAPIOCA FLOUR

Tapioca flour is made from the dried starch of cassava root. It has little flavour, is low in protein and is a useful addition to a wheat-free flour blend. It can be used to thicken sweet and savoury sauces, but the sauce will become a little 'stretchy' and gel-like. It is a good substitute for potato flour and arrowroot. Available in Asian grocery stores and some health-food shops.

XANTHAN GUM (FOOD ADDITIVE 415)

Xanthan gum is a vegetable gum used in baked goods to help provide elasticity and keep them moist. It is a cream-coloured powder made from the ground, dried cell coat of a laboratory-grown micro-organism called Xanthomonas campestris. It is the most common vegetable gum used in wheat-free cooking, though guar gum or CMC can be used instead. Available from health-food shops.

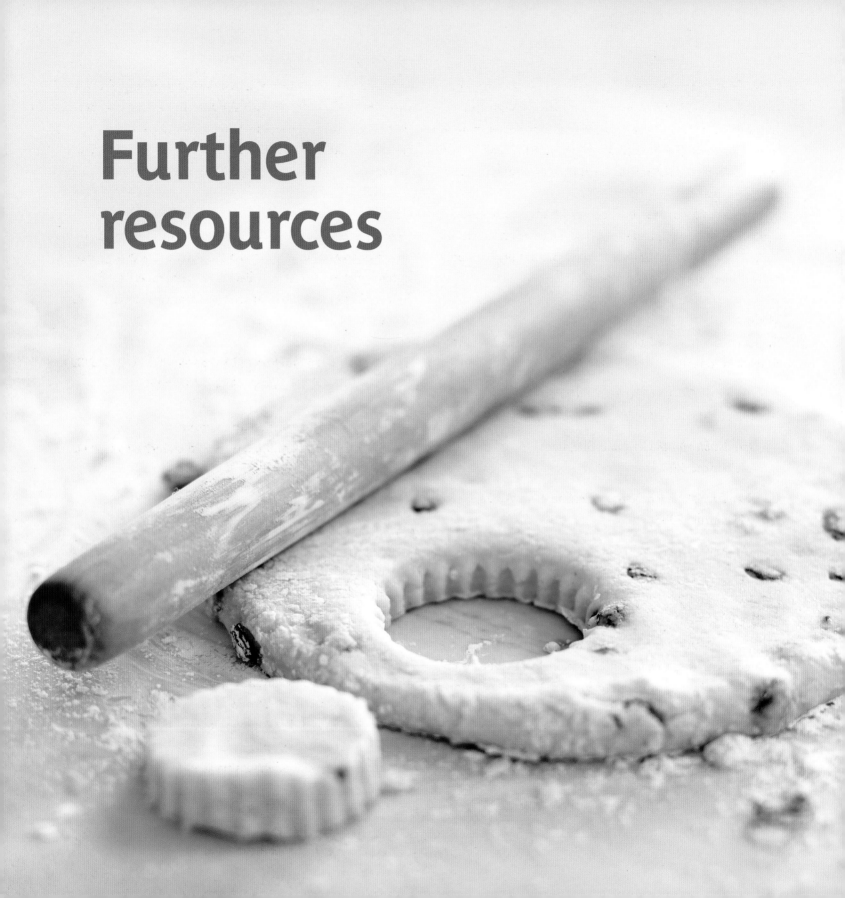

Further resources

THIS BOOK cannot possibly cover all topics of relevance to the Low-FODMAP Diet. Our website, foodintolerance-managementplan.com.au, offers lots of additional information on various topics, as indicated throughout the book. It also contains a list of scientific publications concerning the Low-FODMAP Diet.

In order to follow the Low-FODMAP Diet more easily, it is essential to be equipped with books like this one. Here are some other sources that might help you with shopping, cooking and sharing knowledge.

BOOKS

The following titles by Sue Shepherd are all available at shepherdworks.com.au:

- *The Low FODMAP Diet Food Shopping Guide*, Shepherd Works, Melbourne, 2010.

- *Irresistibles for the Irritable*, Shepherd Works, Melbourne, 2004.

- *Two Irresistible for the Irritable*, Shepherd Works, Melbourne, 2006.

- *Gluten-free Cooking*, Viking, Melbourne, 2007.

- *The Gluten-free Kitchen*, Viking, Melbourne, 2009.

BOOKLETS AND NEWSLETTERS

The Low FODMAP Diet, available at med.monash.edu.au/ehcs

A guide written to support educational workshops training dietitians in how to teach the low-FODMAP Diet to their clients. It also contains recipes.

Irresistible News, subscribe at shepherdworks.com.au

An e-newsletter produced by Sue Shepherd, providing information on gluten-free, Low-FODMAP diets, coeliac disease, IBS and fructose malabsorption. It highlights a range of great gluten-free/wheat-free events, delicious recipes, invitations to take part in research, food and restaurant reviews and more.

DIETITIANS

Several times in this book, we recommend seeking the advice of an Accredited Practising Dietitian. Ask your gastroenterologist or GP about dietitians with expertise in the Low-FODMAP Diet. If they cannot help, you could try the following.

The Dietitians Association of Australia, (02) 6163 5200 daa.asn.au. Search 'Allergy and food sensitivity'.

Shepherd Works, shepherdworks.com.au

Sue Shepherd's dietitian practice offers individual, group and telephone consultations.

RESEARCH

med.monash.edu.au/ehcs

Visit this website for information on participating in or donating to current scientific research into food intolerance and FODMAPs.

FOOD DIARY

Copy the food diary on the next page (or download it from this book's website, foodintolerancemanagementplan.com.au) and use it to keep track of your daily FODMAP intake. You will find it very useful not only to work out which foods cause your symptoms to flare up, but also if you decide at any stage to consult an Accredited Practising Dietitian.

YOUR FOOD DIARY

WEEK _____

DAY	BREAKFAST	MID-MORNING	LUNCH

AFTERNOON	DINNER	SUPPER	SYMPTOMS

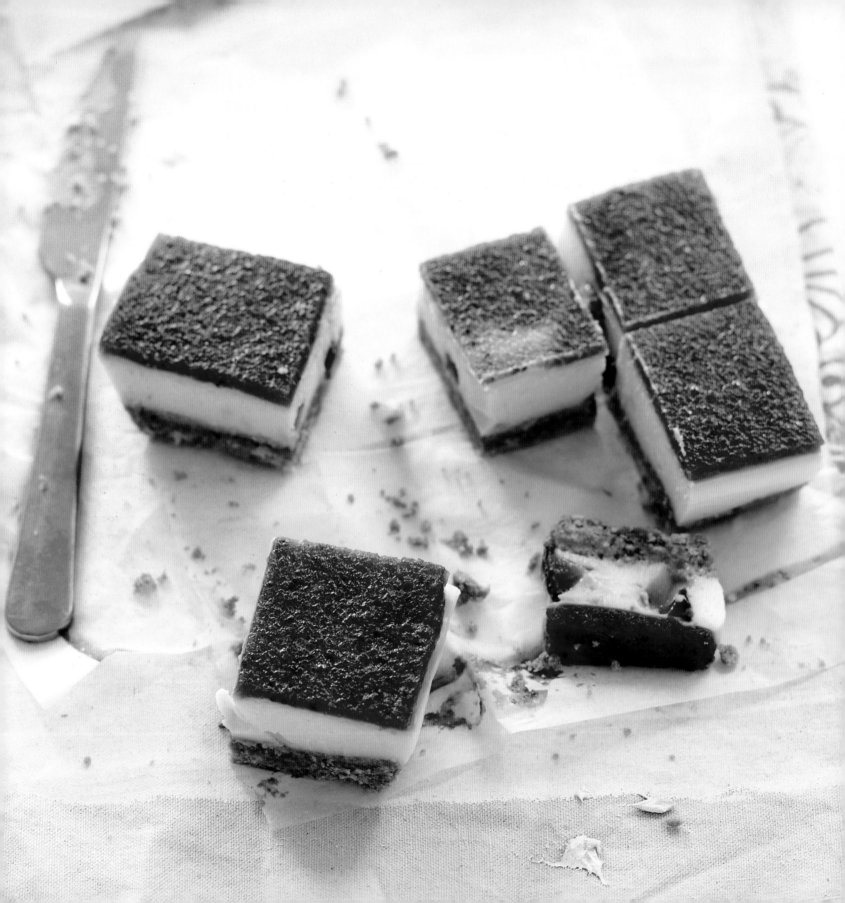

Acknowledgements

IT IS A PLEASURABLE but difficult task to duly acknowledge all of the wonderful people who have supported us on this great journey to introduce our FODMAP concept to the international stage.

Thanks first to our families and friends. Over many years, you have listened to stories of our progress and provided enthusiastic support for each of our achievements. We thank you for sharing it all and know this is as much a celebration for you as it is for us.

To the team at the Eastern Health Clinical School, Monash University: your hard work and diligence in research excellence have helped further develop and realise FODMAP concepts. Your efforts are greatly appreciated and it is a privilege to work with you. Thanks to the dietitians at Shepherd Works, who have helped support the growth of FODMAP research by applying it to so many patients. To all our colleagues who are clinicians and clinical researchers in the Department of Gastroenterology and Hepatology at Eastern Health/Box Hill Hospital: thank you for believing in us. We also thank many medical colleagues outside Eastern Health who have embraced and supported the concepts. To our professional associations, the Dietitian's Association of Australia and the Gastroenterological Society of Australia, we so appreciate your enthusiastic acknowledgment of this innovative therapy. And sincere gratitude to our patients, who provide us with such a sense of purpose, motivating us to do our very best at all times. Thanks also to inspirational foodie friends Jo Richardson, Tobie Puttock, Peta Gray and Spencer Clements.

We are indebted to the wonderful team at Penguin for having confidence in the FODMAP concept, and allowing us to describe it so comprehensively to help improving the quality of life of so many. Thanks to Julie Gibbs and Ingrid Ohlsson for your belief, and Rachel Carter and Nicola Young for editorial excellence. Thanks to photographer Mark O'Meara, food stylist Sarah O'Brien and home economist Tracey Meharg for the mouth-watering photographs, and to Megan Pigott for overseeing the shoot. Thanks also to Elissa Webb for her sensational design.

To the friends, colleagues and acquaintances who have not been specifically mentioned, thank you for your very special role in our lives.

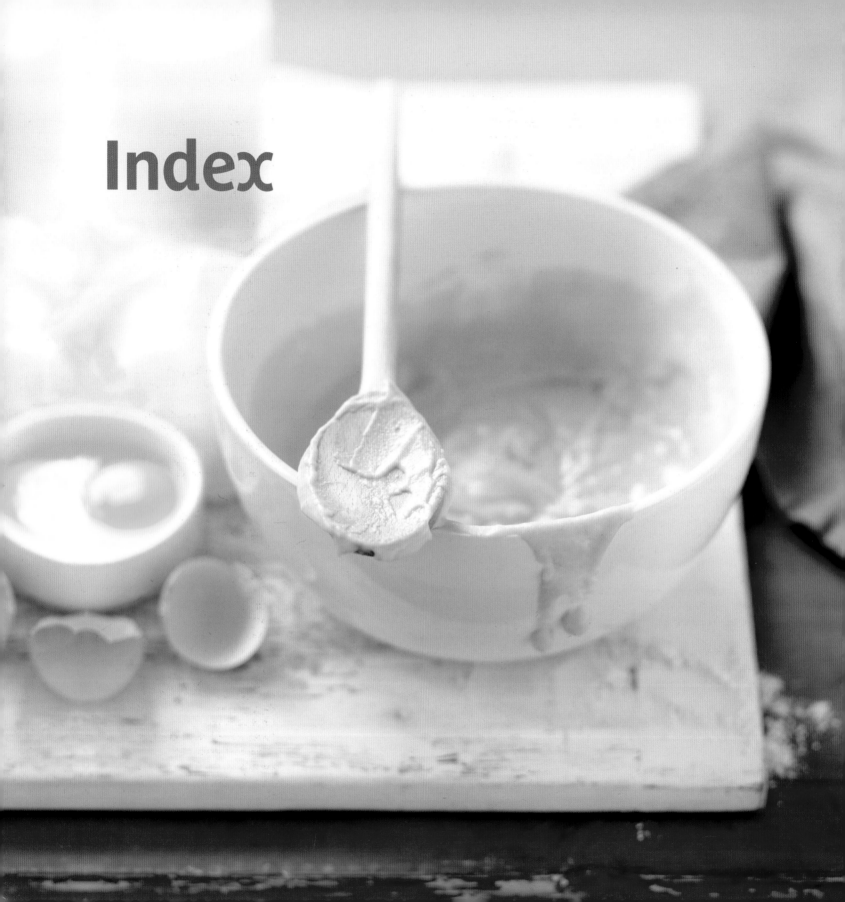

Index

VIKING

Published by the Penguin Group
Penguin Group (Australia)
250 Camberwell Road, Camberwell, Victoria 3124, Australia
(a division of Pearson Australia Group Pty Ltd)
Penguin Group (USA) Inc.
375 Hudson Street, New York, New York 10014, USA
Penguin Group (Canada)
90 Eglinton Avenue East, Suite 700, Toronto, Canada ON M4P 2Y3
(a division of Pearson Penguin Canada Inc.)
Penguin Books Ltd
80 Strand, London WC2R 0RL, England
Penguin Ireland
25 St Stephen's Green, Dublin 2, Ireland
(a division of Penguin Books Ltd)
Penguin Books India Pvt Ltd
11 Community Centre, Panchsheel Park, New Delhi – 110 017, India
Penguin Group (NZ)
67 Apollo Drive, Rosedale, North Shore 0632, New Zealand
(a division of Pearson New Zealand Ltd)
Penguin Books (South Africa) (Pty) Ltd
24 Sturdee Avenue, Rosebank, Johannesburg 2196, South Africa

Penguin Books Ltd, Registered Offices: 80 Strand, London, WC2R 0RL, England

First published by Penguin Group (Australia), 2011

10 9 8 7 6 5 4 3 2 1

Design by Elissa Webb © Penguin Group (Australia)
Photography by Mark O'Meara
Styling by Sarah O'Brien
Illustration on page 6 by Andrea Danti / Shutterstock
Typeset in 11/16pt Chaparral Pro Light by Post Pre-press Group, Brisbane, Queensland
Colour reproduction by Splitting Image Colour Studio Pty Ltd, Clayton, Victoria
Printed and bound in China by Imago Productions

National Library of Australia
Cataloguing-in-Publication data:

Shepherd, Sue.

Food intolerance management plan / Sue Shepherd and Peter Gibson;
photography by Mark O'Meara.

9780670074419 (pbk.)

Includes index.

Subjects: Food allergy – Diet therapy.
Gluten-free diet – Recipes.
Milk-free diet – Recipes.

Other Authors/Contributors:
Gibson, Peter Raymond.
O'Meara, Mark.

616.9750654

penguin.com.au

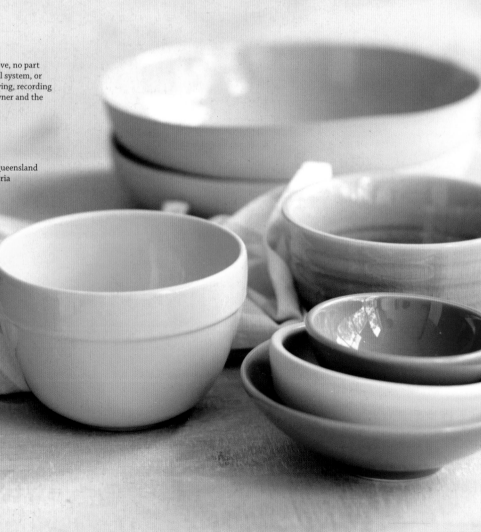